Birthright

by Betsy Dewey

Published by Mom Owners

Published by MomOwners
Visit www.momowners.com

Birthright
Copyright © 2011 by Betsy Dewey.

Published in the United States of America

Cover design © by MomOwners

Photo courtesy of Susie Mickel
Endeavors Photography
www.endeavors.Smugmug.com

Contents

Part I -
Important Things Every Pregnant Woman Should Know

Part II -
Preparing for Baby

Part III -
Tips on Getting Pregnant and
Staying That Way

Dedication

I am a regular American woman. I was raised going to public school and the Presbyterian Church. I went to Vanderbilt University and then on to The University of North Carolina for my postgraduate work.

I have been a linguist, a music teacher, a performer, a massage therapist, a writer, a business owner, and now a mother.

I thought being pregnant and giving birth sounded scary. The stories I'd heard about giving birth in the hospital freaked me out. I thought you were shaven, given an enema, cut from vagina to rectum (episiotomy), given labor-inducing drugs, watched by residents, told what to do, hooked up to IV units, unable to move, and miserable, even after the baby was taken from you and put in an incubator.

I experienced none of these things. And you don't have to either. The aforementioned things are not normal and should never be routine.

Women are by nature intuitive, but many of us don't trust our intuitions.

Learn again to trust what you feel. Learn again to seek It.

Ladies, ladies, please, let's take our bodies back. Let's reclaim birth. Birth is first and foremost a spiritual experience, like death. Walk into birth with courage and love. Let go of fear. You could die walking down the street, but you don't fear it. Yes, you could die giving birth; it's highly unlikely, but true. There's still no reason to fear it.

Reclaim your birthing experience. Love it. It is your own, and it is the one thing that will connect you with all of your mothers and their mothers and their mothers. Dare to give birth your way.

If the idea appeals to you that pregnancy and birth can be a beautiful, exciting, and sacred rite of passage that honors the mother and the new life within her, this book is dedicated to you.

As you'll soon figure out, I do most things as naturally as possible. When I give pointers in this book about homebirth, breastfeeding, etc. please keep in mind that every child and every situation is unique. I don't know why, but my experiences so far have been good and relatively easy. Perhaps it was because my children were born at home with no intervention. Perhaps it's because I read every book I could get my hands on. Perhaps it was because I had access to the wisdom of midwives. I don't know.

This book is my two million cents. Never let anything or anyone make you think there's something wrong with you or your child or your birth. I've written this book simply to help educate my sisters. This is for you.

Acknowledgements

I send out a HUGE thanks to the following people. I couldn't have gotten the book here without you:

Becky Shatto, Susie McCartney Nelson, My-Cherie Haley, Stephanie and Ben Labay, Kayla Hoffman, Laura Mire, Melanie Shatto, Emma Rose Anderson, Leigh Anne Graf, Marimikel Penn, Debra Day, Ilyssa Foster, Aleah Penn, Tree Dewey, and Bon Crowder. And if there is anyone else who read the manuscript and gave me feedback whom I am forgetting, I apologize.

I am eternally grateful to Dr. James Vance and Lynda Shannon, my beloved chiropractor and acupuncturist respectively, for the loving care that I received from before I conceived to this day. I know for sure that you both had a lot to do behind the scenes when it comes to me being a mom. Thank you, more than I can say. I love you both dearly.

Also, I am grateful beyond words to my beloved husband. You have taken this path with me and championed these natural choices from the start. I remember when you said that the book should really be for men because if men out there knew this stuff, they'd never let their partners give birth in a hospital. Thank you, my love, for everything.

And Miss Sonya. Thank you. Your friendship and time has been priceless. I cannot possibly express my gratitude enough.

Preface

Over the years, I have noticed that no matter what kind of lifestyle and habits a woman may have on her own, some powerful influence overtakes her when she learns of a new life growing within. All of a sudden, there is a desire for pure, whole, and natural.

She understands that her health choices are now affecting the most vulnerable and innocent. She feels a sense of "ownership" for something that is only hers, yet also the world's. And she wants to tend to her "responsibility," her "gift" well. Somehow, she is newly inspired to eat well, exercise, read and research, and live fully aware – especially when the luxuries of time and peace of mind are afforded.

But, oh, how much information is now readily at our fingertips! More than we have time to sift through, it seems. *Birthright* is perfect because it filters and condenses the most valuable information about pregnancy and childbirth in an inspiring and practical way.

Betsy's writing is real and honest. She is passionate and has great conviction about that which she has known most personally. Her energy is contagious, even through pages of a book.

Birthright is for every woman who is pregnant or seeking to be pregnant. This book will shed light on facts you might not have been aware of, in hopes that you will not tread lightly into your decision about where to give birth. I have three children of my own, and even though I traveled a more "natural" route with my pregnancies and deliveries, I know I would have done things differently had I known more of what is in this book, *Birthright*.

Birthright has long been in the making. A trail of special women have left their mark through their support and feedback. I have been a lucky one to come in during the final stretch and cross the finish line with them all. It is our hope that many women will be inspired and informed by Betsy's gift – to live more naturally, to birth "right," and hope of hopes, to have their precious babies at home.

Many blessings,

Sonya Dalrymple

Editor

Introduction
Why Every Woman Needs a Midwife

I never knew I needed a midwife. It sounded like something out of Gone With the Wind.

The turning point in my experience as a woman on the planet was witnessing the homebirth and midwife delivery of my nephew. Until then, I thought, as I'd been trained to think, that birth should happen in the hospital. Seeing the birth of Makena at home with friends and loved ones, the midwife masterfully slipping the cord from around his neck, not one, not two, but three times, suctioning his nose and mouth and then coaxing him to breathe, I was forever changed. It was one of the most deeply spiritual experiences of my life. How I wish that birth were something that we all experienced! I knew from that moment forward, any child of mine deserved that kind of reverent birth. The expectation of the midwife is nothing other than a holy, sacred, beautiful birth.

I still didn't know I needed a midwife. I didn't know until I found myself on the brink of a miscarriage. I called the only midwife I knew – the one who had delivered my nephew. She talked me through the miscarriage. Wow. Later she asked when my last "well woman" exam had been. I told her that it had been a while. She said that I really should come in for one, so I did. What I experienced at my exam was totally unexpected.

I loved it. I loved my gynecological exam. My midwife spent a whole hour with me, something that a doctor had never done. There was no exam table; there were no stirrups. It was so natural and unweird. You're on a bed – the same bed in her birthing center that women can choose as a venue for giving birth if home won't do. The midwife just has you slide to the edge of the bed, put the soles of your feet together, and she then kneels on the floor to complete the exam. She asked me when my last eye exam was. She made sure that I flossed my teeth because they've found a link between the bacteria that thrive beneath the gum line and eventual heart disease. She asked me how much I exercise, and what my diet was like. She told me to do Kegel exercises daily so that I will not only have great sex, but also I'll have good bladder control as an older woman. She asked how my emotional life was. In a nutshell, I felt like I had really just had a well-woman exam, from one woman to another.

Within moments of giving birth, my midwife taught me how to breastfeed my newborn by shoving way more of my nipple in the baby's mouth than I thought possible, and voila, he was a champion piglet. She taught me how to avoid mastitis, or a breast infection, by nursing in all different positions, which ensures the emptying of all of the milk ducts. She taught me to not give up on breastfeeding in those first few challenging days by telling me that my baby was on a mission from God to bring in my milk, and that it could take a few days. I stuck with it and nursed whenever my son cried. I had an abundance of milk until we weaned two years later.

My midwife's the one who told me to make sure to stay horizontal in bed for two to four weeks after the birth of my child so that my uterus would heal correctly, and so I probably won't ever need to have a hysterectomy.

She's the one who taught me about elderberry syrup, a natural antiviral you can use to treat flu or take prophylactically to avoid a virus if the people around you have one.

She taught me how to snort salt water when I think I'm getting a sinus infection.

And on top of all the things about which she's raised my awareness, she made my pregnancy and birth so easy, so predictable, so magical, so mine.

Thank you, Marimikel Penn, Debra Day, Ilyssa Foster, and Aleah Penn. There's nothing like having true wise women around when you need them.

They enlightened me in so many ways. Every woman who gives birth – at home or in the hospital – should have access to all of the information I was so lovingly given during my pregnancy. So here's this book. If you don't have access to a midwife (geographically, financially, or even legally in some states) this book is my gift to you. In it, I've tried to compile all of the information that I learned from my midwives, which is an almost impossible undertaking, considering I can't translate their wisdom and friendship into words. I have, however, done my best.

May our children be born with reverence, gentleness, and love –

Betsy Dewey

November 2008 – June 2011

Part I

Important Things
Every Pregnant
Woman
Should Know

- Chapter 1 -
How to Have a Healthy Pregnancy: Rules to Live By

I learned many juicy tidbits from my midwife about having a healthy pregnancy. Here goes:

Do Kegels daily.

Doing Kegels daily is imperative. 200 of them a day in fact. Yes, do them now, and do them all the time. If you don't know what they are, they're basically vaginal weightlifting. You find the muscle group by tightening the muscles you would use to stop peeing in mid-stream.

Just tighten, hold, and release about 20 times. By strengthening the pelvic floor muscles now, you will stretch and avoid tearing during delivery. Strong muscles stretch. Weak muscles tear.

When you're not pregnant, keep doing Kegels, and you'll always be sure to have rockin' good sex. And do you expect to still be continent as an older woman? Depends. Depends on whether or not you've done Kegels all of your life.

Exercise almost everyday.

Walking is crucial. Swimming is awesome. Yoga is sublime.

You need to be in really good shape when you give birth. *The main reason for transport to the hospital during a homebirth is exhaustion.* Your legs, arms, and core muscles need to be strong, so you can endure hours of contractions and squats. Another reason to exercise regularly is that exercise oxygenates the blood of both of you, and this makes for a very healthy little tyke.

Back in the day, women were constantly squatting and walking. Getting exercise wasn't something they had to make themselves do. I say this because I truly believe that women's bodies are meant to give birth. If you don't exercise a lot during your pregnancy, you might really have trouble giving birth naturally. You might lack the strength. But then again, you are a woman, and you might just rock. My midwife, however, berated me about the exercise, and she knows what makes labor easier.

Swimming is really the ideal pregnancy exercise due to its low impact, full-body workout, and positional benefit to the baby. And just a head's up – if you haven't swam laps in years, it's really a booger at first. Just do as many as you can, add a few each time, and in two weeks you'll be amazed at how many laps you can swim before you're pooped.

If you can't or don't want to swim regularly during your pregnancy, then you need to be doing the tabletop pose for 20 minutes every day for the last trimester. Just get down on your hands and knees, *belly down*, and wiggle. This is important because the baby's spine needs to come around to the front of your body. Ideal birth position is head down and spine out in front (anterior). The spine is the heavy part of the baby, and gravity is our friend.

And the flip side – don't lie on your back on the couch. It has the opposite effect of swimming and the tabletop pose. It puts the baby's spine beside your spine, and that's not a fun way to give birth. It's called "back labor." The baby's hard, bony parts are against your hard, bony parts in the birth canal, and it's harder and more painful for both of you.

When lying around, lie on your side, and preferably the left side as it increases blood flow to the placenta.

Don't run.

Your ligaments and connective tissue are being softened by a hormone called relaxin when you are pregnant. It allows your pelvis to open up and give birth. If you run or do any high-impact exercise when you're pregnant, you risk messing up your joints. Even yoga should be done with care, preferably in a prenatal yoga class. You can easily over-stretch when you're pregnant.

Drink a gallon of water a day.

This keeps your baby's amniotic fluid, as well as your liver and kidneys, as flushed as possible. The amniotic fluid where your baby swims around is also where she pees and drinks. If you are well-hydrated, then so is your child. Also, you are eliminating for two (not just eating for two).

You'll know this by the intense flatulence that sometimes accompanies pregnancy, and you can blame it on the baby. But seriously, by being well-hydrated, you will encourage the healthy elimination of toxins and both of your wastes via your liver, kidneys, intestines, and skin. As an aside, drink the majority of this gallon early in the day. If you're trying to get it in just before bed, you'll pay for it with numerous trips to the potty while you'd much rather be sleeping.

Take your prenatal vitamins and minerals.

I feel like everyone knows this, but it must be included in any chapter such as this. Folic acid is crucial to the proper neurological development of a fetus. Calcium and other minerals are fundamental as well. If you aren't consuming enough calcium, the baby's developing system will leach it from your bones. Both of you need it. Omega 3,6,9 is the other supplement that insures healthy brain development. Some people swear that fish oil makes your baby smarter.

Make healthy smoothies

A fabulous way to get a big, natural dose of good stuff everyday is to have a smoothie for breakfast.

Here's a recipe:

1 cup Almond Milk

1 scoop Protein Powder

1 scoop Green Vibrance (or other "green food" powder)

1 organic frozen chopped banana

1 cup organic frozen fruit

1 tsp. Ground flax seeds

1 T. organic coconut oil (super health food!)

Blend until smooth. Drink for your health!

- Most items can be found at your local health food store.

- If you haven't previously peeled, broken, and frozen any bananas, you can add a cup of ice and a regular banana to get the same effect. However, frozen bananas make for a great consistency. Toddlers love them too!

Remember this smoothie throughout your life whenever you're feeling low on energy.

Carry healthy snacks with you at all times.

A significant drop in blood sugar, also known as "morning sickness," can happen at any time of the day. The reason it usually happens in the morning is because right when you wake up, you usually haven't eaten in eight hours.

To keep it at bay, eat protein right before you go to bed, and eat something highly nutritious when you wake up to pee at night. I did this religiously this second time around, and I can't even begin to tell you how much better it was.

Have a sandwich in the fridge at all times and a protein bar in your nightstand. Right when you wake up, eat some yogurt or something else that's easy, and then go make breakfast. When you're pregnant, you need to eat something nutritious every two hours or so, to keep from having a blood sugar crash that makes you want to wretch. There are lots of really nutritious, good bars out there these days. Lara Bars have no refined sugar. Kind and Luna bars are also good. Protein bars might become your best friend. Just EAT!

Make sure that your relationships are healthy.

If you and your partner are fighting, it's time to get some counseling. If you're depressed, ditto. Your mental health is just as important as your physical health when it comes to the development of your child.

Floss your gums daily.

Be sure that you're flossing your gums everyday. The bacteria beneath the gum line has been linked to heart disease and other ailments. There's no telling what that nasty stuff could be doing to your developing child.

Dwell on positive news and ideas.

Turn off the news or anything else that's scary or negative. If you get worried or afraid, you produce neurotransmitters associated with these feelings. These icky chemicals circulate into your baby, and then she feels worry and fear for no reason. You need to feel good. You live in the most affluent society ever in the history of mankind. There is plenty for everyone. Live a life of gratitude and joy. If you listen to crap, then you'll attract crap. Keep all of the music, TV, movies, people and energy in your life positive. If you haven't owed it to yourself yet, you at least owe it to the little innocent within you. A person's personality begins in the womb.

Here's one last rule to live by when you're pregnant:

Don't stand when you can sit.

Don't sit when you can lie down,

and don't just lie down when you can sleep.

~ Chapter 2 ~

The List: Other Things I Learned from my Midwives

As I write this, I realize how important midwives are. They are so beautifully educating such a tiny percentage of American women about how to give birth. Not only that, but they are also raising awareness about so many pertinent issues that are facing women today whether we know it or not.

Since the 1970's, when midwifery came back to life in the U.S., midwives have been the ones on the front lines of advocacy for women and babies all over the world. They are the ones who have fought for breastfeeding in developing countries where contaminated water and formula kill babies. They are the ones who, through education, have helped us let go of the fear of the intact penis and brought the circumcision rate down from 85% to 56%. They are the ones who have fought for a baby's right to eat in public. They are not alone. There are plenty of nurses, doctors, and other men and women who have joined these causes, but it's the midwives who are on the front lines.

My purpose in writing this book and in speaking to women is twofold. One, I want women to know about the reverent option of homebirth. It's such a gentle and loving way for a child to make the transition from the womb to the world. Two, if you don't choose homebirth, I want you to know everything I learned from my midwives so that at least you'll know how to give birth.

The ideas in many chapters of this book were introduced to me by my midwife such as the stages of labor, cloth diapers, home made baby food, and birth plans. This chapter lists all the other things I learned from her.

Before Labor

Oil your belly

There are many oils to choose from these days that are specifically for moisturizing your stretching skin during pregnancy. I made mine from a base of almond oil with a few drops of rose and patchouly essential oils. Be sure that you oil your belly, hips and breasts from the first trimester on. It really helps with stretch marks.

Dr. Christopher's Prenatal Herb Capsules

You start taking these herbs six weeks before your due date: one a day the first week, two a day the second week, and so on. These herbs help your cervix soften so that labor is just a little easier.

Omega 3,6,9 Oils

Great oils to take on a daily basis include fish oil, evening primrose, black currant, flax, or a 3,6,9. The best thing would be to cycle through them. These nourish you baby's brain and soften your cervix.

Castor Oil Packs

You get some castor oil, put a little on a soft cloth and heat it. Make sure it's not too hot! Put it up against your perineum and sit on it for 20 minutes. Do this daily for the last month of your pregnancy. Castor oil softens the perineum and helps it to stretch.

Perineal Stretches

This one is no fun, but anything you can do to ease birth and avoid tearing is worth it. You can't do it yourself, so you get your partner to lube up his finger with pure vitamin E oil and gently place it into your vagina up to the middle knuckle (about 1.5 – 2 inches) and press down on the perineum. He makes a "U" shape as he runs his finger from side to side doing the stretch.

It sounds fun, but it hurts. But you're just stretching what will stretch much more than that when the baby comes. Do this daily for about a month before your due date.

Note: I did all of the above suggestions, and I still had minor tearing of the superficial skin layers upon delivery of my baby. Why? Perhaps it was because I pushed so well that my midwives had not had the time to put warm olive oil compresses on my perineum. I was being rushed to have the baby, and I was still in the squatting position when my son arrived. You have more tears when the actual birth takes place in squatting position.

Perhaps minor tearing is pretty normal. My midwife thinks it is. By minor, I mean superficial tearing of the skin on the outside of the perineum. My midwife sewed up my tears, and there is no trace today that I ever tore.

Serious tearing involves the actual musculature of the perineum. I would imagine that the Kegels, castor oil packs, herbs, and perineal stretches kept serious tearing at bay for me. When you have an episiotomy, when they cut the perineum during labor, they cut through these muscles. After being sewn together, muscles take a long, painful time to heal.

Episiotomy is still fairly routine in the hospital, but it is a controversial procedure because sometimes they cut accidentally all the way into the rectum, and sometimes you end up with an infection. In a nutshell, it is unnecessary surgery/intervention that can cause more harm than good. Minor tearing is normal and tears heal well. I recommend doing everything you can to keep major tears from happening and skipping the episiotomy.

During Labor

The Sleeping Trick

This is one of the most amazing things I learned from my midwife. It's a way to actually get valuable sleep toward the beginning of labor. You can have labor pains for several days before the actual birth. Contractions can be twenty minutes apart for a whole day and then stop for a day or two before real labor begins. In any case, if your contractions are still more than ten minutes apart, and it's between 9 PM and 4 AM, you need your sleep! You've got to have your strength when the big day arrives. Here's what you do to "trick" your body into stopping contractions long enough for you to get a few hours of sleep.

You take two ibuprofen, a glass of red wine, and a hot bath. That's it. That's the trick. Your smooth muscles will relax, and you'll be able to sleep. It's heavenly. I did this two nights in a row. The night before I gave birth I slept for about 3.5 hours. We called the midwives about 3 PM the next day, and I gave birth at 8 PM.

Here is a caveat – if you are really into the stages of labor and birth is eminent, if you do the trick, it will not stop labor. On the contrary, it brings it on!

Move

And you simply have to walk around during labor – move, move, move! Giving birth is literally nothing you can do laying down! Squat, stand, walk, sing — you get the idea. This allows labor to really come on so you won't "need" intervention

Post Labor

Lie Down After Birth!

The most important thing to know after the birth of your child is to stay in bed, literally horizontal, for a minimum of two weeks. Most western women are unaware of how important this is. After birth, your uterus weighs about 4 pounds and is the size of a baby. Over the next twelve weeks it will return totally back to normal – about 4 ounces and the size of your fist. The majority of this healing takes place in the first two weeks. If you are up and about, you risk something called a prolapsed uterus and will likely need a hysterectomy in your 50's.

You need to lay flat so that your uterus will heal properly. You can raise up on your elbows to eat (the food that someone else has prepared for you and brought to you.) Nurse your baby sidelying. And only get up to use the restroom and shower. You can only be up for 10 minutes a day.

The hardest part of this is receiving. You will find it very difficult to do. Have a bell by your bed so you're not constantly shouting for something. Have a gallon of water, food, and plenty of diapers within reach. And enjoy being the queen in bed with your tiny angelic heir/heiress for maybe the best two weeks of your life.

Afterease Tincture

For a few days after birth, your uterus is going to continue contracting in an effort to return to normal. It hurts. You don't have all of the hormones helping you with pain that you had during labor. So you get this herbal tincture called "Afterease."

You can find it or something similar at an herb shop or online. (I found mine at www.wishgardenherbs.com). Every time you have a postpartum contraction, you just take a dropper full, and voila the pain goes away. It worked like a charm for me.

For the first few days, every time your baby latches on to nurse, the hormones rush signals your uterus to contract. This is a good thing and another reason to breastfeed. It was like clock work: bite bullet, latch on, dropper full of afterease, bliss.

Sun and Sitz Baths

If you have stitches after birth, sit in an herbal postpartum sitz bath 2-3 times daily to cleanse and to draw blood to the area to promote healing. It's suggested that you don't submerge yourself in a regular tub until you're done healing.

You can find the dried herbs already prepared in muslin bags at herb shops and on line. Also try to sun your stitches everyday until they heal. You'll need a private backyard or rooftop for this one.

Sun Your Newborn

This is counterintuitive, but we did it, and our newborn stayed super healthy after his birth. You hold your newborn directly in the sun's rays in the morning or afternoon if the weather is warm, or through an open window if the weather is cold, for 10 minutes everyday, five minutes on one side, five minutes on the other. This keeps the child from developing jaundice, which is caused by the inability of the baby's immature liver to break down red blood cells, leading to an increase in the level of bilirubin in the baby's blood. Sun your baby for about a week. It works like a charm.

Goldenseal Powder For the Cord Scab

Buy a small amount of goldenseal powder at your local herb shop. Two or three teaspoons will be enough. Clean the cord stump really well with a cotton ball and alcohol. After a few days you can really bend the stump around and really get in there. Use a fresh Q-tip and dab some of the powder on and around the umbilical cord scab twice a day until it falls off at about 10-14 days old. It encourages healing by keeping it dry and clean. The standard procedure calls for the use of alcohol only. Moms who have used both swear by the goldenseal, stating that the umbilical cord has fewer problems and falls off faster. Both of my boys' cords were problem free using this method.

Arnica

This is the most amazing stuff – seriously. It makes bruises go away. I first learned of arnica from the mother of a five-year-old who had slammed his hand in a car door the day before. She immediately put topical arnica gel on his hand and had him take the homeopathic arnica sugar pills. The next day, no one, not even the boy himself, could tell that anything had happened the day before.

My own experiences with this homeopathic medicine are no less impressive. The sooner you use it after an injury, the more effective it is. It is for bruising, muscle trauma, and pain. You do not use it topically if the skin is broken. My midwife covered the bruises from the birth canal on my newborn's head with arnica, and they were gone the next day. I took a few pills after giving birth to ease all of the muscle exertion.

From the smallest bruise to major trauma, arnica is nothing short of miraculous. I keep both the pills and the gel in my diaper bag. My whole family uses it, but especially my toddler. Buy it at your local health food store.

Newborn Fingernails

Newborn fingernails are as thin and sharp as paper, but you can't cut them with clippers because they are still attached to the skin of the finger underneath. My midwife taught me to bite the edge of the finger nail and to pull sideways and up at the same time, effectively tearing it off. At first this was counter-intuitive, and I thought I might hurt my baby. It is quite the opposite. I bit and tore off my newborn's fingernails for months and never hurt him once.

Important Information

My midwife gave us a "Birthing Packet" when we signed on for her services. This packet included pages on nutrition, heartburn, indigestion, constipation, cloth diapers, water birth, how to obtain a birth certificate, backache, supplements, anemia, yeast and bacterial infections, herpes, hemorrhoids, varicose veins, self breast exam, breastfeeding benefits, breastfeeding basics, mastitis (breast infection), the newborn bill of rights, mother-infant bonding, cesarean section, what to hand a hungry toddler, lactation nutrition, birth kit order form, child birth classes, midwifery, my midwife's education, certification, and services. There was a lot more than that to boot. It was indeed quite a volume. I still refer to it to this day.

There are two pages that I feel compelled to share with you in full because it is information that every new mother should have access to. I have included them with permission from my midwife, Marimikel Penn.

16

Call Us Immediately If

- There is water leaking from the vagina

- There is any bleeding from the vagina (a little touch of pink or red is not necessarily abnormal, especially after sex, serious exercise or a long day on the feet, but call anyway)

- Illness i.e. Sinus infection, bladder infection symptoms (burning, stinging, or an urgency when peeing) stomach flu, respiratory infection symptoms, food poisoning

- Bad fall

- Severe emotional upset

- Car wreck

- Regular contractions before 37 weeks that are getting longer, stronger, and closer together

- Vaginal infection

- If you just need to talk

Weird But Normal Things With Your Newborn Baby

- Broken blood vessels in the whites of the baby's eyes

- Blood in the urine. It can be spots of blood or a peachy color.

- Spitting up blood, especially if the baby was suctioned

- Xyphoid Process at the end of the sternum may protrude

- Sneezing and coughing

- At around 4 weeks, the baby can get baby acne

- White dots on the nose, milia

- Their eyes wander, sometimes in different directions.

- Hands and feet are bluish in the first 24 hours after birth

- Baby spits up

- Mom may have broken blood vessels in face and eyes from pushing hard

- Mom may have a fist size clot. Multiple fist size clots however are not normal and you should call the midwife

- Blisters on the baby's lips (from nursing)

- Peeling

- Feet curved (massage them, lengthen the tendons)

- Shuddering

- Eyes roll back

Not normal things include:

- Grunting exhales

- Color changes, especially blueness

- Not nursing

- Lethargy, difficulty rousing.

- Serious yellow skin

- Chapter 3 -
Normal Birth

I know that sounds weird – normal birth, but read on . . .

Natural birth just means you did it without drugs.

"Normal" means you were lucky enough to give birth intuitively – just plain ol' normal birth with no intervention at all.

Unbelievably, this is a new concept for the western world. Well, it's not exactly new. It's how all women gave birth until we forgot how. So, it's not new. It's lost and being recovered. The basic idea is this: **If the mother and baby are both doing well, leave them alone.**

This is a tough one for most doctors and midwives because usually when you're getting paid in our society, it's for *doing* something. Even midwives, who typically advocate natural childbirth, meaning birth without drugs and medical interventions, still jump in there and start telling you to push just as soon as you're dilated to 10 centimeters.

Are they doing their job if they just stand back and let birth happen normally? Dogs, cows, cats, horses, monkeys, walruses (you get the picture) — *every single other species of mammal in the world just gives birth*. No one is telling them to push. If the mother and the baby are both doing just fine, perhaps the best job a birth attendant can do, would be to simply let it happen. Let the woman keep on giving birth instinctually. I love the idea.

There's even an idea coming around that even when a woman's cervix is fully effaced and dilated, maybe she doesn't need to start pushing. There can be a moment to rest at this point. There are situations when the baby might even come on out on its own.

In my first case, however, it probably wouldn't have worked like that. My midwife's keen focus allowed her to recognize that every time I lay down, my baby's heart tones went down. She deduced that when I lay down, something was compressing the umbilical cord and compromising my baby's oxygen supply. She therefore required me to stay upright the whole time I was dilating from 7 to 10 centimeters. I pretty much just sat on the toilet lid. Then I was on hands and knees when I needed to push. My midwife kept saying, "Come on sweetie, you need to go ahead and have this baby." We were a long way from the hospital, which in hindsight, might have been a good thing.

It is very possible that if I had gone to the hospital, at some point, someone, a nurse on duty, a doctor, or a technician, would have recognized the low heart tones but not the cause of them, and would have suggested a C-section. After all, a lack of oxygen to the brain of a baby can lead to cerebral palsy or far worse. Fortunately, my midwife had a keen sense of observation and a whole lot of experience.

I needed the help of a pro at the birth of my first son, so technically I didn't have a "normal" birth, but it was an entirely natural one at home, and it was the best day of my life. With the birth of my second son, I unwittingly got to experience what this chapter is about. Since the midwife didn't make it in time, I got to *just give birth*, and it was amazing. Once again, the best day of my life occurred. I love giving birth.

How do you have a baby if no one is telling you what to do? *You* get to decide.

Move Around

One of the single most important things that a laboring woman does is move around. You get up, walk around, you squat, you hang by your hands, you sit, you wiggle around on all fours. The last thing you want to do is lie down. This is one of the biggest differences between hospital and home birth. Every woman I've interviewed who gave birth in the hospital was told to lie down during most of the time she was laboring. I'm sure there are exceptions to this rule; I just haven't run across them. Moving around keeps things moving, literally. Being upright, walking, squatting, and hanging all use gravity to help your baby out. Moving also takes your mind off of labor, even if just for a moment.

With my second labor, I was moving around until the birth was imminent because I didn't even know I was that far along. I had read an awesome book called *Active Birth* by Janet Balaskas during my second pregnancy. She corroborated what I had been encouraged to do during my first labor by my midwife – MOVE!! It makes the birth happen faster.

This doesn't mean to go out and walk 10 miles to kick in labor. The last thing you want is exhaustion. In fact, for the last two weeks before your due date, you really want to take it easy – no more than 4 hours of work a day. Once you realize that labor is in full swing, get moving!

Eat and Drink

During a normal birth you are encouraged to drink **plenty of water each hour**. Coconut water is one of the best things you can sip on. It replenishes you like nothing else, and it's totally natural.

You are encouraged to eat if you're hungry. You need the energy.

My midwife just told me to eat only things that I wouldn't mind seeing again. Nausea during childbirth is totally normal and not something to be avoided by not eating. However, it is recommended that you not throw up if you can help it. If you start to feel nauseous during labor, someone needs to put cool wet rags on your forehead and neck.

Homebirth

If you're planning to have a normal or natural birth, you need to plan to have a homebirth. It's almost unheard of to have zero intervention in the hospital, and it's counterintuitive for the hospital staff to stand there, do nothing, and just wait for your baby to come. They want to "help your labor along," and give you pitocin, a chemically derived pseudo-oxytocin. How the heck are you going to roll around, hang and squat with an IV needle in your arm? Your own body knows more about birthing your baby than anyone else. It produces a massive rush of oxytocin when you need it. I'll take my own, Nature-made-by-way-of-my-endocrine-system drugs, thank you very much.

Hospital Birth

Here's the typical scenario for a hospital birth, even if you're planning to do it naturally:

They let you labor (in between vitals checks) until they can't stand to watch you or listen to you anymore. After all, most hospital staff has never seen (or heard) a totally natural childbirth, so they offer you something to "take the edge off." DON'T DO IT! You need that edge which your own endorphins have kept at bay. If they give you a painkiller, your endocrine system will quit producing the natural ones, and when it wears off, you're in more trouble than you were when you took the drugs.

It's a great idea to put a pretty sign on the door that says something like,

Natural Childbirth in progress:

please do not offer any drugs or intervention.

Enter only if you are totally supportive

of this family's decision.

They might offer you pitocin to "speed things up a little." Again, DON'T DO IT!! What you don't know is that when pitocin "speeds things up a little," it also intensifies the pain. So, even if you declined the drugs the first time, you're pretty much going to be begging for them after the pitocin. So, you've started down the slippery slope of passive, unempowered birth. After your epidural, your labor slows way down (because you can't feel anything anymore), "fails to progress," and might even stop. They then tell you you've been laboring too long and that you need to have a cesarean birth. What they don't tell you and don't even know, is that if they had left well enough alone, you'd have a drug-free, alert baby in your arms already, and you'd be able to get up and pee by yourself!

I simply must include here that my midwife has a hypothesis that pitocin could be partly involved in the recent increase in autism. There is no science to support this yet, but she's noticed that the rise in the use of pitocin parallels that of the rise in autism. She thinks that the drugs we use during labor and birth might interfere with the bonding process that occurs when only the body's own natural hormones like oxytocin are involved. When we were talking about this, I asked her how many of the children of whom she had attended birth had been diagnosed with autism. She looked me in the eye and said, "None that I know of." She has attended the births of over 3000 babies. If extrapolated against the 1 in 150 statistic, 20 of them should be autistic.

I Didn't Know I Was Pregnant

Lately, I saw a cable TV program called "I Didn't Know I Was Pregnant." Yes, it sounds absurd, but apparently the stories of these women are true. During labor, which was baffling to these women, two of them actually delivered their babies in the toilet without even knowing it, and one fell out onto the bathroom floor. Think about that. Having a lower abdominal urge to push, they naturally went to the toilet. They then pushed a baby out, felt relieved, and walked away. (No mention was made of the umbilical cord.)

This leads me to believe that first of all, if you don't know you're having a baby, it's apparently that easy. I didn't know I was in labor with my second baby, and it *was* that easy.

Second of all, you need to be upright, squatting, or on all fours to make labor a snap. All of the other women in the show ended up in the hospital because they were having intense contractions but didn't know what was going on. In one lady's case, the staff couldn't even figure out that she was pregnant and in labor. All of them were made to lie down when they were pushing. This is so counterintuitive. Each hospital staff was in a frenzy looking for what in the world was going to be wrong with these babies when their mothers had just been going about their business for nine months instead of taking vitamins and avoiding fumes, cigarettes, and alcohol. All of the babies, even the set of twins, were perfectly healthy.

I've never given birth in a hospital, and after seeing that show, I hope to God I never do.

I just want to give birth, nothing more, nothing less. Normal.

- Chapter 4 -
Labor

Giving birth was the most amazing thing I've ever done. It's nothing to fear. Sometimes we're the poet goddess. Sometimes we're the garden goddess. Sometimes we're the business, school, or teacher goddess. We take on these roles with ease. Why would we want to numb ourselves to the greatest rite of passage that we will ever experience? The question stymies me. When you are pregnant, there is no question that you are the goddess, growing new life inside you. So put on your goddess birthing robe and walk into the most amazing experience that you will ever have. Labor.

Understanding the different stages of labor that you will experience helps prepare you to confidently embrace this rite of passage.

Warm-Up Labor

Warm-up labor describes the contractions that begin in the hours or days before true labor comes on. Some people refer to labor that seems to begin and then stop as *false* labor. I don't use this term. Warm-up labor can take several days or just a few hours. It's characterized by contractions that come and go.

Stages of Labor

The stages of labor are as follows:

- Dilation (labor) usually takes 6-12 hours

- Pushing and birth of the baby usually takes 1-2 hours

- Birth of the Placenta usually takes 5-15 minutes

- Getting your uterus back to normal usually takes 12 weeks

- Nursing – the longer the better

Dilation

The *phases* of labor (all of which occur during the first stage of labor) are as follows:

- Pre-labor (doesn't stop like warm-up labor)

- Early labor (from 1-4 centimeters) is the longest part.

- Active Labor (from 3-7 centimeters)

- Transition (from 7-10 centimeters) is usually the hardest and shortest part.

Typically, these phases of labor are characterized by certain feelings. During pre-labor, there are often feelings of discouragement. Discouragement that there's a long way to go, and that you haven't dilated that much yet. Early labor is usually characterized by a feeling of excitement that it's really happening. Active labor's characteristic feeling is one of seriousness. At some point during active or transitional labor, the warrior takes over, and you just want to get it done. Transition can be both an altered state of consciousness and discouragement.

The magical hormones that are released during transition are delightful. Not only do they help to get you through the process, but they also punctuate the sacred quality of giving birth. It can even be trippy and psychedelic at this point, which for me was quite pleasant. I personally remember transition as my favorite part of labor. It didn't seem like the most difficult phase because I was so filled with the spirit of a warrior. If you have an epidural, pitocin, or a cesarean birth, I'm quite certain that your experience of transition will be altered, and I feel like you'll be missing out. In fact, I can say for certain that my unaltered experience was phenomenal and something that I'd want all women to experience. It's something that only women can experience, and I'd never take that away from anyone.

Honestly, the short, magical time from transition to holding your baby in your arms is probably what's driving me to write this whole book.

Pushing

I remember a woman who was talking about giving birth. She said, "Push like you're taking the biggest dump of your life." Ladies, if you push like that, you'll push the lining of your rectum plumb out. This is how you end up with hemorrhoids for life. You're not taking a dump. You're pushing a baby out of your vagina. If you don't want bloody eyes and hemorrhoids after childbirth, listen up.

There are five things to remember when it comes to pushing.

1. Make your body into a "C" shape.

2. Breathe in all the way, then let out 1/3 of the breath. Hold 2/3 a breath and push.

3. Don't make a sound.

4. Push like it's a "reverse Kegel." (like with your vagina –
NOT like you're pooping.)

5. Use your abdominal muscles to push in and down.

If possible, be upright or on all fours in order to really use your contractions and gravity.

The "C" shape means to tuck your chin in to your chest. You let a third of a breath out when you push to avoid pushing with a full breath. Pushing with a full breath is what causes women to break the blood vessels in their faces and eyes.

The "reverse Kegel" is really hard to imagine if you're not pregnant. But if you are pregnant, for some reason it makes sense. Do a Kegel. Now, as you release it, tuck your chin to your chest and release slowly, pushing in and down with your stomach muscles. There it is, the reverse Kegel, and that's what pushing should feel like.

I compiled all of this info before giving birth, and I kind of pushed a little too well. My midwife said, "Okay, Sweetie, just give me one more good push, and we'll get you up on that bed and deliver the baby." So, I gave the mother of all pushes, and my baby just shot out right then and there, giving me four superficial tears. Usually, the baby's head is born on one push and then the shoulders and body come on the next one. But my son came out all in one push.

Every birth is as unique as the two individuals involved. Some women experience a huge urge to push. Some women never need to push at all.

I don't remember an urge to push. I just remember the sense of urgency that I go ahead and have the baby, considering that his heart tones were low when I was on my back. I pushed him out without really having taken the time for him to crown properly or

29

having given the time for the midwives to lube me up with warm olive oil. So, I tore, not badly at all, and my midwife just sewed me up right then and there.

Considering how healthy my baby turned out, I wouldn't change a thing. I'm glad I pushed, and I'm glad he shot out.

Just give birth. It's really very simple. And exciting. And fun, exhausting, riveting, joyful, monumental, and beautiful.

Birth of the Placenta

The birth of the placenta is a snap and usually happens pretty quickly after birth.

Something you might look into are the health properties of consuming your placenta after you give birth. I can't speak from experience, but I know that people have it encapsulated or will even make it into a smoothie soon after the birth. Your midwife will know more about this if it interests you. If you don't have a midwife, find a local one who will come make the capsules for you. You can also give your placenta back to the Earth. If you have a home birth, you get to decide.

Contraction of Uterus

After the placenta comes, the uterus naturally begins to contract. It will do this for approximately the next 12 weeks. I can see why they call this the 4th stage of labor as your uterus is still busy, busy. This is a time for you to rest. *Especially for the first two weeks* you simply must stay down – **horizontally**. My midwife's theory on preventing a prolapsed uterus by allowing it heal properly resonates loud and clear with me.

Nursing

I also see why this is considered a stage of labor. It's simply amazing how connected the uterus and the breasts are. Every time your sweet little angel latches on to nurse those first few days, you immediately experience a post-partum contraction, and that's good! So, I wonder if it means that I'm still laboring just because I'm still nursing my 20 month old. Hmmmm.

- Chapter 5 -
What Do Midwives Do?

In French, a midwife is called "sage-femme" or wise woman. There are numerous reasons for this. In some parts of the world, their techniques have been handed down without interruption through countless generations of women.

Chapters 1 and 2 list the sage advice my midwife gave me during pregnancy. This chapter spells out what they actually do.

I've seen many talented musicians and athletes who were in the "zone," but never one as impressive as my midwife. I chose my midwife because I saw her deliver my nephew. That day changed the course of my life forever and was the initial domino leading to this book.

How unfortunate it is that we don't witness birth anymore. People used to be there when their sisters, mothers and neighbors were giving birth. It's such a normal thing, and it's nothing to fear.

When my nephew was born, the unusually long umbilical cord was wrapped around his neck three times and his head was blue. It didn't look good. Without hesitation, she masterfully slipped her finger under one wrap of the cord and slipped it over his head. Everyone in the room was holding their breath as she repeated the move two more times. She then turned him over in her hand and started rubbing him vigorously on the back saying, "Come on, Baby. Come on, Baby." She turned him face up and suctioned off his face, nose, and mouth, turned him back over again and rubbed again. He gasped, his head turned pink, and we all breathed. He was here. I knew in that instant that if I ever had a kid, she would be the one to bring him into the world.

And she was! She was one of the most professional individuals I've ever worked with, and I've never received better care in my whole life, aside from that of my own mother. From my first gynecological exam to the last of the postpartum home visits, I was in the hands of someone whose entire focus was the health of my baby and me.

My midwife taught me how to give birth which makes her job a lot easier. In fact, she made it so clear that I was the one with the hard job. I was the one giving birth. She would be there only to assist. A midwife is like a wedding planner. Between the two of you, many hours are spent to make sure that the event goes off without a hitch. Attention is given to every detail. When there is a hitch, she unhitches it.

Pregnancy Visits

My midwife spent a minimum of 45 minutes with me at every office visit. Sometimes it was even an hour and a half. She always asked me if I was exercising, what I was eating, how my relationship with my husband was, and if I was doing my 200 Kegels a day. She counseled me on my weight gain and my emotional health every time.

She also did all of the things you'd expect at a doctor's office. She checked sugar levels in my urine to make sure I wasn't developing gestational diabetes. She checked my blood iron level. She listened to the baby's heartbeat. She weighed me. She measured my belly to make sure I was on track. As I got further along, she'd feel the baby and tell me his position.

Childbirth Classes

She offered seven mandatory two-hour childbirth classes. They were mandatory for both the expectant mother and her birthing partner. I learned oodles of information during these 14 hours.

My husband and I felt entirely prepared for the birth. In fact, after the class on what to do in case of "sudden child birth," which is where it happens so fast that the midwife doesn't even have time to get there, I asked my husband if he felt like he could handle it. He said, "100 percent."

In hind-sight, that was a really good thing. The birth of my second son was so "sudden" that the midwife didn't make it in time, and my husband had the honors. He, his sister, and my mom helped me pull it off on my own. *And I **loved** it – giving birth on my own.*

At each class we watched a birthing video. After seeing seven natural births, just plain ol' giving birth the old fashioned way, I felt so at ease with it. I almost wasn't afraid at all.

Labor Preparation

About three weeks before my due date, my midwife made her first house call to my home. She wanted to be absolutely certain of the route to my house in case she got the call in the middle of the night. She familiarized herself with my house and how I wanted things at the birth. She made sure that my bedroom was set up the way she had asked. (She needs a cleared table and to have room to pull the makeshift "hospital room" out of her bag.)

My midwife taught me when to make THE CALL, and this is of huge importance. You aren't really in bona fide, dilating labor until your contractions are no more than five minutes apart with each one stronger, longer and sooner than the last one. She referred to this as "stronger, longer and closer together."

Women typically have pretty intense contractions for a few days before birth. They can even get going and then stop for a day.

If you're having a homebirth, you want your midwife to show up for the delivery well-rested. If she shows up too early, she won't be at her peak at the time of delivery. If you're going to the hospital, and you show up 27 hours early, you end up having a "27 hour" labor.

My husband called the midwife when the time came. She showed up 40 minutes later, which was remarkably fast considering how far out of town I live. When she arrived, I was one centimeter dilated. Five hours later, I was a mother.

Thoughtful Details

Aside from the education and postpartum home visits, my favorite thing about midwives is what they do at your house during and after the birth. When my midwife and her apprentices showed up at my house, one of them immediately came back and got me off of my bed. She said, "Go walk around, eat and drink if you want. We've got to get your bed ready."

As I had been instructed to do, I had two sets of sterilized sheets ready for them. You sterilize them weeks in advance by putting them into paper grocery sacks and placing them in the oven with a pan of water on the bottom rack. You bake them at 250 degrees for an hour, and voila, you have totally sterile sheets in a totally sterile bag. They took the sheets off of the bed. They then put the "postpartum" set of sterile sheets on the bed. They covered them with a sheet of plastic, and covered the plastic with the second set of sterile sheets, the "birth" set.

After you give birth, they scoot you and the baby over to one side of the bed and start removing the birth sheets and the plastic sheet. You and the baby scoot over to the waiting set of sterile sheets, and they whisk the birth sheets off to your washing machine where they get every drop of blood out with hydrogen peroxide. My super clean house was even cleaner after they left.

The midwives cooked food for themselves and for my family while I was laboring. They even fed my dogs. They let me be alone with my husband for the majority of the labor, and only came to me when I was in need. They did come in now and then to check the baby's heart beat with a fetal monitor. When I dilated to seven centimeters, the midwives never left my side.

~ ~ ~ ~ ~

My midwife had taught me how to give birth, the stages of labor, and everything to expect. She taught my husband how to encourage and help me during labor. She had taught me how to push. For the duration of labor, she took impeccable birth notes, which document the entire birth. She then presented me with them upon leaving. Within 15 minutes of the birth, she showed me how to breastfeed. And the reason it took that long was because right after the birth, she was busy injecting me with local anesthesia and sewing up my five minor tears.

I can't speak highly enough to do the process justice. It was the best day of my life, and it was all because of the wedding planner, I mean midwife.

Postpartum Visits

I would have thought that it all ended there, but my midwife's attention had practically just begun. Twenty-four hours later, then on the third day, the fifth day, the seventh day, she showed up at my house again to check on me and the baby. **I cannot express the importance of the postpartum home visits enough.**

It seems luxurious, but the fact is that it is life saving and should be a part of every woman's postpartum care. Postpartum hemorrhage is life threatening.

Ina May Gaskin, American homebirth pioneer, wrote an article for *Mothering Magazine* (March-April 2008) entitled, "Masking Maternal Mortality." In it she describes the fate of six very different women. One was a single mother who was found having bled to death in her apartment from a hemorrhage. Her newborn had also died from dehydration and starvation. Another woman was a married mother of three who died in her husband's arms. Three died after the cesarean births of their first babies.

For a birth professional, postpartum hemorrhage is easy to recognize and easy to treat. It is inexcusable. In countries with very low maternal mortality rates, like Australia, England, the Netherlands, New Zealand, Norway, Scotland and many more, trained nurses make home visits in the days following birth.[3]

Another major point of Ina May's article is that of our wonderful 50 states, only 21 of them ask a question for the death certificate that has something to do with whether or not the deceased was pregnant or had given birth in the weeks preceding her death. In other words, we don't even have accurate maternal mortality statistics in the USA. Ina May raises the question of, "Why is no one talking about this?"

I left my house once during the month after the birth of my son. That outing was for the 2-week baby and mama visit to my midwife, and we also stopped at the chiropractor to have both the baby and me adjusted after the birth. It was the best month of my life.

My midwife required me to stay in bed for at least two weeks to let my uterus heal. Your uterus, which normally weighs 4 ounces and is about the size of your fist, weighs 4 pounds after birth and is the size of a baby. In 12 miraculous weeks, it will return to normal. If during those first two weeks you're up and around, you risk needing a hysterectomy later in life due to a prolapsed uterus. That's basically when the poor thing kind of caves in.

Women have to recover from childbirth. During my obligatory two weeks in bed, I could only get up to use the bathroom, to shower, and to take my herbal sitz baths to help heal my stitches. In other words, I was treated like a queen who had just given birth to a king. I'd relive those two weeks over and over for the rest of my life if I could, sitz baths and all.

At my six-week check up at my midwife's office, I cried. I was really sad not to be seeing her anymore. She had been my pillar, my teacher, my healthcare provider, my sister, my drill sergeant, and my friend. Pregnancy just might be the most spiritual time in a woman's life. It's certainly one of the most magical times, and I had shared all of it with her. I still see her once a year for my "well woman" exam, which I love.

Anticipated Cost

The whole experience – the monthly checkups through month 6, the twice monthly checkups until delivery, the child birth classes, the home delivery and postpartum home visits, plus every phone call I ever made to ask about anything, and access to the lending library – all cost $4500.

Some midwives charge a little more, some a little less, and many midwives have a sliding scale so that they can accommodate all kinds of women. The bottom of my midwife's sliding scale is her cost – $3000. She couldn't do this for everyone, or she couldn't stay in business.

I understand that some insurance companies are starting to cover midwifery, which makes a whole lot of sense for everybody considering hospital births can cost as much as $30,000.

Some women who want homebirth are still stuck with hospital births because their insurance will only cover hospital birth, and they can't imagine paying their insurance premium as well as paying for a midwife out of pocket. If we start choosing insurance companies because they cover midwifery, they'll all get on board.

- Chapter 6 -
Home Birth:
The Safe, Fun, and Spiritual Way to Welcome Your Baby to the World

Imagine this. You're about to experience one of the single most magical days of your life.

Instead of going to a room you've never been in, with people you've never seen before, you find yourself in your own room surrounded by familiar faces. Anyone you want to be there with you can be. You have your sweet music playing. You have candles lit. Your pets are there. You slip in and out of your own warm bathtub. You walk around, naked if you want, by that time you're tired of your clothes. It's fun. You sing and make the noises of a female mammal preparing to give birth. The spiritual nature of birth, whatever that means to you, is unhindered. You don't care who can hear you. You walk around your yard or down the street if you want. You come in and rest for a minute on your couch. You call a friend. You kiss and lay with your husband. You do some yoga. You make sure someone is taking pictures.

You have your baby. The midwife places her on your belly and she starts immediately to nurse. The emotion you feel is indescribable. The lights are dim and the welcome music for your child is playing. The feeling in the room is overwhelmingly spiritual in nature, similar to when someone is dying. The miracle of life, contact with the great unknown, and union with the spiritual world has just taken place. The placenta comes, and your partner cuts the cord if he wants to do so. The midwife shows you your placenta and asks what you want to do with it. She and her apprentices help you to get cleaned up and put the room in order. No one ever once takes your baby away from you without your consent. No one gives your baby a mandatory vaccination. You never get in a car. You spend the night at home . . . with your baby.

The memories of birthing at home are yours forever – that cedar branch you hung from during contractions, the look on your mom's face as she stood at the door of your bedroom watching her grandson crown, that exact place on the floor where your baby was unexpectedly delivered.

This is homebirth.

I never would have thought that you could have your baby at home; I'm the fourth of four children happily born in the hospital. Homebirth would never have crossed my mind, except that I got the rare chance to see one. Considering how much I like to avoid hospitals, I was immediately enthralled. I don't even want to die in a hospital. The only reason you'll catch me in a hospital is if my life needs to be saved. If I'm just doing something that doesn't require a doctor, like being born or dying, I'd like to be with friends and family.

More Safe than Medical Error

Anyone who thinks that homebirth is dangerous is totally uninformed. Birth is inherently a tiny bit risky. No matter where you give birth, there is a very small chance that you or your baby could die or have complications.

In our country, you have an 8 in 100,000 chance of dying during or right after childbirth. [4] Statistically, both maternal and infant death are higher in hospital births than in homebirths. Interventions in the hospital such as drugs, epidural, c-section, episiotomy, forceps use, vacuum extraction etc. are leading factors in birth complications. These interventions are unnecessary about 93% of the time.

The main risk at home is the miniscule chance that the baby would need life-saving intervention at the moment of birth. The main risks in the hospital are due to the high instance of unnecessary intervention and human error. Every single study shows homebirth to be safer for both mother and child.

~ ~ ~ ~ ~

What it boils down to is this: *giving birth is safe*. There is no reason to fear birthing anywhere. You have the option to do it at home if you want to. If you are at home and your midwife suspects a problem, you will transport to a hospital.

Homebirth is statistically safer than hospital birth, yet less than 1% of American babies are born at home. In a six year study done by the Texas Department of Health, it was found that midwife attended birth has about 1/3 the infant mortality rate of physician attended birth.[5]

In the Netherlands, 34% of babies are born at home with midwives[6], and it stands to reason then that the infant[7] and maternal[8] mortality rates are lower there. In the same way that it's not logical to be afraid of flying since you're more likely to die each time you step into your car than each time you board an airplane, it's not logical to be afraid to give birth at home. We fear the unknown, and that's the problem here. Ninety-nine percent of babies are born in hospitals, which renders homebirth an unknown. You are more likely to encounter a problem or to require intervention when you give birth in a hospital. The reasons for this are numerous.

First of all, childbirth is not a medical condition and should not be treated that way. Medical errors in hospitals cause more deaths than car accidents each year. (See the following excerpt for the reference.) If you are healthy and not dying, you are wise to stay away from hospitals. Hospitals are where sick people go. The hospital staff is looking for pathology and problems. It disturbs me greatly that there are those who insist that hospitals are the only place where women should legally be allowed to give birth. If you give birth at home, you are not at risk of hospital error.

An in-depth study came out in the year 2000 called, "To Err is Human." The following is an excerpt:

> *The knowledgeable health reporter for the Boston Globe, Betsy Lehman, died from an overdose during chemotherapy. Willie King had the wrong leg amputated. Ben Kolb was eight years old when he died during "minor" surgery due to a drug mix-up.*
>
> *These horrific cases that make the headlines are just the tip of the iceberg. Two large studies, one conducted in Colorado and Utah and the other in New York, found that adverse events occurred in 2.9 and 3.7 percent of hospitalizations, respectively. In Colorado and Utah hospitals, 6.6 percent of adverse events led to death, as compared with 13.6 percent in New York hospitals. In both of these studies, over half of these adverse events resulted from medical errors and could have been prevented.*
>
> *When extrapolated to the over 33.6 million admissions to U.S. hospitals in 1997, the results of the study in Colorado and Utah imply that at least 44,000 Americans die each year as a result of*

medical errors. The results of the New York Study suggest the number may be as high as 98,000. Even when using the lower estimate, deaths due to medical errors exceed the number attributable to the 8th-leading cause of death. More people die in a given year as a result of medical errors than from motor vehicle accidents (43,458), breast cancer (42,297), or AIDS (16,516).[9]

If you have what's considered a "high risk" pregnancy, then you might be required by the laws of your state to give birth in a hospital, or you might just want to. Usually women who have health issues are considered "high risk." Women with cancer, diabetes, and other medical conditions and illnesses fall into this category. Women who develop toxemia, preeclampsia, or who have multiple fetuses are also considered "high risk." Breech babies, twins, and moms who are over 40 can absolutely experience birth at home successfully. Your rate of transport to the hospital will be higher, but if you want to be at home, you probably can be. If you're having twins, your state might require that you and your midwife meet at the hospital, but you can still have your babies with your midwife as naturally as possible. My midwife, personally, will only assist with twins at the hospital.

People often compare labor to running a marathon. Indeed, they both require a high level of fitness. People sometimes collapse and need medical attention during a marathon, but that doesn't mean that marathons should be held in a hospital. You go to the hospital if you need to. Labor, like a marathon, can be grueling and deeply spiritual, but other than that, neither of them is all that big of a deal. People do them all the time.

Where are You Comfortable?

I have to stress here that the decision of where to give birth should rely on where you feel the most comfortable, on where you feel the least fear. You must feel empowered by your decision.

Spend some time considering where you want to give birth: home, birthing center, or hospital.

Weigh the possibilities. Even if the idea of homebirth is like a fairytale to you, but you still fear not being in a hospital, go with the decision that reduces your fear the most. If you are scared to give birth at home, then don't. If you're scared of hospitals, give birth at home or at a birthing center. Ideally you'll be at peace with the process no matter where you end up. Fear is not your friend. It would be best to surrender all your fear. Read the chapter on "Overcoming the Fear of Childbirth," watch birth videos (Youtube is a great resource for birth videos including home births), watch "The Business of Being Born," and interview a midwife. If you're still certain that the hospital is for you, then go there and never think about it again. You are no less of a Goddess. Birth is magical no matter where it happens.

I knew that I wanted homebirth long before I was ever pregnant. However, the actual decision was still a significant one for me. We moved 25 minutes away from the hospital where my midwife prefers to transport when necessary. In traffic, make that closer to an hour away.

I believe that what is to be will be. I believed in my body's ability to give birth. I sat down and had a powwow with the little person inside my womb. I could feel that he wanted and deserved to make his grand entrance out here in nature, amongst friends and family, in the reverent environment of our home. I trusted my instincts. I didn't want his first glimpse of the world to be a hospital room. I wanted his transition from womb to breast to be as loving as possible. I asked my baby to guide me. After that meditation, I never questioned our decision. I knew that if everything went great, it would be amazing, and that there are no guarantees. The pros simply outweighed the cons. My husband was entirely in favor of homebirth as well, and having a supportive partner helps to seal the deal.

Do you like eating and drinking what you want to? Do you like your home? Do you like sleeping in your own bed? Do you like making your own decisions? Do you think your body probably knows how to give birth? If you answered "yes" to these questions, you'd probably enjoy having your baby at home.

Whichever decision you make, make it, and don't look back.

- Chapter 7 -
Born in the USA:
Cesarean Section in America

If you don't already know this, you need to. One of every three women who give birth in the hospital in America today will be given a cesarean section. Read that again.

Historically only about 5% of women actually need to have a C-section. "According to the World Health Organization (WHO), anytime a country's cesarean section rate rises above 15%, the dangers of C-section surgery outweigh the life-saving benefits it is supposed to provide."[10] The Netherlands C-section rate in 2002 was just 13.5%.[11] In the 1980's, when the C-section rate rose above 15% for the first time in the US, maternity activists were up in arms saying that any doctor whose C-section rate was above 5% was endangering women's and children's lives. Today, any doctor whose C-section rate is below 15% is considered to have women's best interest at heart. There are many whose C-section rates are over 40%.

Cesarean section is currently the most commonly performed major surgery in the US. Why is this? For three reasons, really. One, some doctors just want to get home for dinner. (Can you blame them when they schedule 40 births a month?)

Two, because of our litigious society. If a doctor gets sued for negligence during the delivery of a baby and he or she has performed a C-section, the "evidence" is pretty clear that he or she did everything in his or her power, including performing major surgery, in order that lives might be saved. The sad thing is that more lives are actually lost as a result of this surgery.

Three, OBGYNs are surgeons. Surgery is what they are trained to do, and they make quite a bit more money when they do it. They are not trained to facilitate natural childbirth.

During a vaginal delivery, the hormonal symphony that allowed you to become pregnant and kept you that way comes to its awesome climax. Hormonal communication between fetus and mom is what causes labor to begin. Oxytocin rushes in and starts contractions. I call it a "hormonal symphony" because that's the best way I can describe it. Everything is so perfect, from the delivery of the child and the placenta, to the milk coming in and the postpartum contractions that heal the uterus. The benefits of this symphony to mother and child are still little known, but if you deliver by C-section, you just don't get them.

Enough sources are ripping up C-sections right now. See *Mothering Magazine*'s September-October 2007 issue or *The Business of Being Born* for more. The *Mothering* article is fabulously informative – including many statistics on safety, and an illustrated play-by-play of an actual cesarean, which you really should check out if you're considering an elective cesarean birth.

My purpose isn't to tear the birth industry a new one; it's to educate women about birth options. I'm so grateful that we live in the best country in the world, especially when it comes to western surgery and diagnostics. If you're one of the 5% of women who truly need a cesarean birth, hallelujah that you're here and probably 5-10 minutes from a hospital where competent men and women are there to assist you at any hour, every day. Amen.

– Chapter 8 –
C-Sections, Inductions and Why You Need a Strong-Willed Advocate in the Hospital

If you are planning a hospital birth, or if you end up at a hospital after transport from home, you are going to need someone there who can champion your desires. In the middle of labor, you are in no position to make decisions that you have to fight for. Your partner, husband, mother, midwife, doula, friend, or someone must be there who knows your wishes and can stand up to an entire hospital staff if need be.

You must know in advance and preferably in writing what you want. Do you want a totally normal or natural birth? Perhaps you don't want a cesarean birth unless death is eminent, and you don't want an episiotomy, but if it came down to it, you'd be okay with certain interventions. You need to think this through and know what you want. If you don't, then these types of decisions about your birth will be up to someone else.

C-Section

I've heard many stories from women who were coerced into cesarean birth right in their greatest moment of fear, and later not only regretted it, but they were angry about it. They were in no position to make the decision at the time. Their husbands or partners weren't prepared for the circumstance either.

I'm not blaming the doctors because I believe they are doing the best they know how given the current state of medicine. They practice defensive medicine out of self-preservation in a litigious society. Bless their hearts, but you need an advocate any time you end up in the hospital.

Induction

There is almost never a reason to induce labor. Due date, shmue date. Western practitioners determine your "due date" from the date of your last menstrual period. They typically assume that you ovulated on day 14 of that cycle. If you ovulated on day 19, like I did last month, your "due date" is already five days too early.

Some women have very irregular cycles. What if you ovulated on day 25? That's eleven more days of lung development that your baby might have needed. And has it crossed anyone's mind that we're all different? In fact, we're all entirely unique – our sizes, shapes, the age at which we started talking, etc. Some babies might gestate two weeks longer than others, and some definitely come earlier than expected. What if your baby is a late bloomer and wants 43 weeks to complete his mission?

Here's a scenario: no one knows it, but your due date is already two weeks early because you ovulated after day 14, and you couldn't really remember the actual date of the start of your period anyway. The due date falls on a Monday, and your doctor is going out of town the Thursday before that. You schedule your birth for the Tuesday before he leaves. The doctor has been "concerned" about your pregnancy since early on when your baby wasn't ever quite where it should be on the growth charts. (He didn't know that your baby was right on schedule for when you actually conceived.) You do what you're told and schedule the induction. The drugs they give you to induce labor don't make the baby come "fast enough." You end up with a cesarean birth. You never know that your baby really needed three more weeks in the womb. You always wonder why he suffers from asthma.

The fetus' lungs are one of the last things to fully develop. On that miraculous day that hormonal communication starts labor, the gig's up. Perhaps the placenta just can't meet the demands of the fetus anymore. Perhaps the lungs are so ready to breathe air or the belly is so ready for milk . . .no one knows what gives the green light, but what we know is – that's when it's time, it's time. You can't make the sun rise any earlier than it's going to. You can't make a seed sprout before it's ready. You can't make winter go away. If you could, you'd mess everything up. Unfortunately, you *can* induce your baby before it's ready. Why anyone would do this for any other reason than to save a life, I'll never know.

There are reasons to induce the baby if it truly is far overdue, but nearly every woman is given pitocin in the hospital to "help labor along." If you want to give birth the way women have for 400,000 years, you're going to have to have someone in the hospital with you running interference.

A Strong-Willed Advocate

I know a woman who just wanted to get up during labor. She was in the hospital, and thought it was just wonderful that they were letting her husband in the room with her. Hospitals had come a long way since her first birth in the 1970's when fathers weren't allowed in the room. The hospital staff was confining her to bed, which is most unnatural when laboring.

Her doctor was unavailable, and so a substitute came in, introduced himself, and proceeded to give the woman a nickname because he couldn't pronounce her name.

The woman and her husband were so peeved at this point, that when the doctor left the room, they put a chair up against the door. She got up, walked around, and gave birth naturally right there in the hospital. She loved it so much, that she became a midwife and had her next three children at home.

I'm not suggesting you lock your doctor out of your hospital room. I am suggesting that you have someone at the hospital with you who'd be willing to do so in a pinch.

- Chapter 9 -
Interview Some Midwives

Even if you are pretty dang sure that you want to have your baby with a doctor in the hospital, I still recommend that you interview some midwives. What do you have to lose? It's usually free, and you will come away from any hour spent with a midwife as a more empowered and knowledgeable woman.

When you're interviewing a midwife or a doctor, here are some poignant questions to ask:

- What is your C-section percentage? Vacuum extractions? Forceps use? (these should be under 10%)

- What is your induction percentage? Episiotomy percentage? (these should be under 10% too)

- What do you consider to be legitimate reasons for performing a C-section?

- Do you schedule births, or are you willing to be available to deliver on the baby's time schedule? (In other words, will you let the baby come naturally, according to the hormonal dance between mother and baby? Or are you going to induce me so you can get home for dinner?)

- Do you support and encourage natural childbirth? Are you okay with the idea of normal childbirth? (In other words, as long as things are just fine with both mother and baby, are you willing to just stand there and do nothing?)

A few more questions to ask:

- Approximately how many births do you attend per month? (the fewer, the better)

- Do you provide your clients with any birthing classes as part of your services?

- Are you willing to attend homebirths?

- Are postpartum home-visits part of your service?

If you are pregnant and have the misfortune of living in a state like Missouri, where midwifery is considered a felony, you might consider moving to a state where the witch hunts were over 300 years ago and where midwives are held in great esteem, or you really need to contact your Congress people to ask for some new laws to be passed within the next 8 months or so.

Or I suppose you could have an entirely unattended homebirth, but I don't recommend it. Even in our free country, if you live in Missouri, North Dakota, South Dakota, Utah, Illinois or Indiana you're going to the hospital, honey. And at the hospital, there's a one in three chance that your child will be "from his mother's womb untimely ripped." (A reference to the birth of Caesar, hence the term Cesarean Section, from Shakespeare's Macbeth act 5, sc. 10, l. 15-16).

Birthing Centers are becoming more and more popular as alternatives to hospitals. It's possible that even in those states where midwifery is illegal, that you could find an open-minded doctor who offers a birthing center option. This doctor is more likely to encourage natural childbirth and to perform fewer C-sections.

~ Chapter 10 ~
Fetal Testing Does Not Put an End to Your Fears

If you're wondering whether you should have a ream of tests done on your fetus, you're not alone. It's something almost every pregnant woman considers.

My friend, Rachel, is married to a surgeon. His immersion in western medicine required that they test for about 30 different fetal anomalies. So, when I was pregnant and considering all of this, Rachel asked me one thing and told me one thing. They were both invaluable to me.

First of all, she asked, "If you find out that anything is wrong with the baby, are you still going to have it?" If the answer is "yes," then don't bother taking invasive, expensive tests.

Amniocentesis is when they stick a long, big needle right through your belly to get some amniotic fluid. Unfortunately, this procedure can pose a greater instance of risk than some of the issues they use it to test for! For example, Down Syndrome is one of the genetic anomalies that can be detected by amniocentesis. The risk of miscarriage due to amniocentesis is 1 in 200-400.[12] The chance of having a child with Down syndrome is typically 1 in 700-800 depending on your source (and age). For young women, the risk is around 1 in 2500. At age 32, the risk goes up to about 1 in 725, and at 42 the risk is about 1 in 67.[13]

The thing that Rachel *told* me is what I really want to tell you. It's something you couldn't think of from this side of the fence. She said, "Betsy, if you're the fearful type – fearful that your baby might not be "normal" or that something could be wrong, then no amount of fetal testing will put that fear to rest. If all of your tests come back normal, there are still numerous things that they can't test for, and your baby can still get leukemia at age two. *There's always something you can fear if you want.*"

Wow. Now there's a feather in the cap of Surrender. Life is life. It doesn't always smell good, and it certainly isn't always perfect. Let's just relax, let it be, and love whomever the stork has in mind for us.

I'm personally appalled at the number of abortions of Down Syndrome children. Apparently the statistic is very close to 90% of those tested.[14] Who are we to say we are superior to any other type of human being? Down Syndrome children, from all I gather, are extremely special. Their forte is loving. I've heard it said that they are our love teachers here on the planet. Research the subject – what parents of DS kids have to say, how parents feel after the abortion, and anything else you can think of before you even test for Down's. The current trend among doctors, Hitlerian and disturbing, is to recommend the test, and then to recommend abortion if you test positive.

I have a friend who was told she was carrying a Down Syndrome child, and went on to have the baby. Her daughter does not have Down Syndrome. I wonder how many mistakes have been made.

Make your own decisions.

- Chapter 11 -
Overcoming the Fear of Childbirth

Fear of giving birth is totally natural. It's always the unknown. Our minds have been filled with visions of women in the past dying during childbirth. Death during or soon after childbirth (maternal mortality) was a legitimate concern historically. It's not so much the case anymore in developed countries. As I mentioned before, our chance of being one of these statistics is 8 in 100,000.[15] It's much higher than that in developing countries, but you're here.

Overcoming fear is pretty straight forward, and it's downright easy if it's about something that is inevitable. To overcome any fear:

- Stop and think logically.

- Surrender. (Trust the Universe)

- Walk right in.

Fear is usually an illusion. Most fears we experience are of something illusory, something that's not even real or happening. For example, some people have a fear of snakes or spiders that is so bad that they won't even touch a rubber one. Here is something they could try:

- Stop and think logically. This is just a rubber snake.

- Surrender. Due to the harmlessness factor in this scenario, there is nothing to surrender.

- Walk right in. Touch the snake. Your fear evaporates.

This is the treatment used in the psychology world to treat people who have fears that are debilitating to their lives. They call it "exposure therapy," and we could all use a dose. A life lived without fear is a joyful one.

Fear is petrifying. It causes us to shut down and stop really living. FDR was 100% correct in his assessment that, "The only thing we have to fear is fear itself." Haven't you heard that what we visualize over and over we create? It's been called the "law of attraction" lately. Refuse to visualize what you don't want to happen. See only what you do want to happen.

When that rattlesnake is just a foot away, that's when fear is our friend. It signals our autonomic nervous system to heighten our awareness, which just might save our life. But when you're fearing something that isn't actually happening, you're crippling yourself.

Giving birth, like death, is inevitable. There is no reason to fear it. It's just going to happen.

- Stop and think logically. From the dawn of human history, every woman in your lineage (your mom's mom's mom's mom etc.) gave birth successfully, or you wouldn't be here. Birth is something we do. You were born to do it. It's safer now than ever.

- Surrender. If you believe in God or some version of the Divine, then trust It. Hand over your fear. You are deeply loved. In fact, you are love. You are a part of nature. Just as the deeper workings of nature govern the seasons, the tides, and the sunrise, so they govern birth. Don't fight it. Become one with all of the glory of nature that ever has been.

- Walk right in. You have no choice.

My own mother quotes a Bible verse that says, "Perfect love casts out fear."

One thing to know is that contractions aren't hurting you. At any other time in your life, when you experience pain, it's to let you know that something is wrong. Contractions, though, are *helping* you push your baby out. They are intense, but don't fight them. Go with them. Don't fear them. They're not harming you. You are going to be fine, my dear.

Raven Lang, author of *The Birth Book*, wrote,

> *Birth is the strongest force a woman normally experiences. If there is harmony with this force, your body and mind will enter into a different state, one that surrenders totally to natural forces. The face loses self-consciousness; it is a quiet state, gentle and profound. Sometimes I think the ease of a birth has to do with complete surrender to nature, and acceptance of being part of something greater than the individual self, like a beautiful spring, or the first heavy rains, or the sounds and rhythm of the sea.*
>
> *Labor and birth are a matter of believing, trusting, and listening to your instincts – a matter of getting close enough to yourself and to the information you are receiving from your body. You must rely on yourself. You cannot rely on anyone else, a coach, teacher, mate, etc. They are not receiving. I do not mean to de-emphasize the importance of coaches during labor. I simply do not think that they can do it for you, because they can't. Their support and love vibrations are invaluable and make it possible for more than just yourself to share the most beautiful act of love, the joyful bringing forth of life.*
>
> *Tune into labor. Unfold your inherent birth knowledge. Use your own rhythm, get behind it, and don't have your mind in any time dimension except the present. Don't slip into the past, and don't rush into the future. Accept each contraction one at a*

time just as you accept the sun rising each morning, without question, one day at a time.

A factor in labor is the intense sensation. It is beyond the expectation of anyone who has never given birth. This intense sensation is simply a part of the whole, and when there is no fear, it simply is. It is nothing more, nothing to be afraid of, nothing to waste your time and energy fighting against.[16]

Listen to meditations on pregnancy and birth. They will help to evaporate your fear. Get excited about giving birth. It is one of the only rites of passage we experience as women. It alchemizes you. You are going to know that you can do anything after giving birth. Your husband or partner will bow down before your majesty afterward.

~ Chapter 12 ~
The Perception of Pain

In preparation for my second labor, I did some reading on the perception of pain. What I found changed my perception of my own pain, and I honestly felt very little of it during labor.

First of all, labor pain, in the great scheme of pain, is not that big of a deal. These days, humans don't experience pain like people in the past did. We can kill it. Numb it. Never feel it. So it's a shock when we do feel it. Real pain, the kind that won't go away, is what you experience when your arm is crushed or when you have a toothache. It's constant and agonizing.

Labor isn't like that.

Take One Contraction at a Time

Up until the final bit you have 5-20 minute breaks between the pains, which only last less than a minute each time. 30 seconds of pain, a 7 minute rest. 46 seconds of pain, a 5 and a half minute rest. 40 seconds of pain, a four minute rest. It comes in waves, and some are more intense than others. Take each contraction as it comes, and just breathe through that one.

As mine got more intense, I would tell myself, "I just have to get through this one." One in five I had to breathe through.

Learn Breathing Techniques

You should learn and practice some breathing techniques. There are basically two types: fast breathing and slow, deep breathing. Pick what works for you, but you won't know what works for you until you're in labor.

Friends and family were arriving at my house for the birth just hours prior to it, and I was playing hostess. I remember my mom arriving, and I was showing her to the room she'd be staying in. When we got there, I had to stop and put my arms down on the bed. I told her to hold on a minute, and I deep breathed until the contraction passed. I went on to tell her where she could put her things and how happy I was to see her.

When my friend and sister-in-law arrived, once again I was all smiles between contractions. No one, including me, thought I was in real labor, but I absolutely was. Like addicts have to think "one day at a time," when you're in labor, just take one contraction at a time. Before you know it, you'll be in transition when the heavy duty warrior hormones kick in.

Use Contractions to Help Progress

Another trick is to use each contraction to open yourself up like a flower bud. Your cervix has to OPEN to let your baby out. Don't fight the contractions. Use them. Visualize your cervix opening and your baby making headway. Pardon the pun.

Persevere Through Doubting

During both of my labors I reached a point that I call "The Doubt." I reached it right at 6 centimeters during my first labor, and it was about an hour before delivery during my second. (I don't know how dilated I was.) "The Doubt" is when you think you can't do it anymore. You're tired, really tired, and you wish it was over, and you think or say, "I can't do this anymore." Your partner just needs to remind you that this feeling means you're getting close. He needs to tell you that you and the baby are doing a great job and that you're both perfect.

A different kind of pain happens right when the baby is about to crown. I've heard this described as the "ring of fire." It's like a burning sensation as your cervix opens to it's fullest when the baby is actually presenting. You are SO CLOSE to it all being over at this point that you don't really care. You are ecstatic, sweaty, exhausted, and READY. This is when you push the baby out.

Understand Pain in Labor

I can't tell you that birth isn't painful. It is. But it's nothing you can't handle. My midwife shared this wonderful tidbit with me: every other time in your life when you've experienced pain, your body has been telling you that you've been harmed in some way and to stop it. Labor is not that kind of pain. It's good pain, productive pain. Your body is not being harmed by this pain. It's a pain you simply must endure in order to bring forth life. *No pain, no baby.*

I arrive at the conclusion that we only feel the amount of pain that we *think* we are in. As with everything else in life, perception is everything. If you think you are still a day away from giving birth, you just breathe through. If you don't even know you are pregnant like in that silly TV show, you just deal with it and eventually go to the hospital.

Your expectations mean a lot. If you think that labor is unbearable, horrific pain, then it will be. If you think that you can handle it like all your grandmothers did, then you'll do fine. I must admit that the second one was easier, possibly because I knew what to expect, possibly because the way was already paved, or a combination of both. I looked forward to experiencing my second birth. I wasn't afraid at all. Since I really knew it was something my body could do, I looked forward to being there and doing the work with my baby.

You are woman. You are, therefore, inherently a badass. You can give birth. You can love giving birth.

- Chapter 13 -
Visualize Your Ideal Birth and Practice Affirmations

What would your ideal birth be like? Really. Think about it. Dream it. Write it down. Is it in a hospital, at home, at the beach? Who is there? What music is playing? What are you wearing? Are there candles and soft light? Are you meditating, relaxed, and in the zone? This is called your **birth plan**. *Anyone attending your birth should be given a copy.*

Every day it's nice to visualize the beautiful unfolding and surrender that is your birth. Take a few minutes, maybe at bedtime, close your eyes and feel it. Especially visualize the outcome: a peaceful, happy, healthy baby and mommy, smiles, tears of joy, a perfect newborn in your arms. Something that helped me to do this was a meditation CD called *Journeying through Pregnancy and Birth*, distributed by WomanWay. (See Appendix A).

Also take the time to visualize birth the way you *don't* want it to happen just once or twice. This way, you'll have prepared ahead for the worst, and no matter what happens, you'll be okay with it. For me, this was being wheeled down the corridor of a hospital on a gurney, hooked up to an IV, and ending in a cesarean birth. It would all be good, no matter what. For some, it might be having the baby suddenly in a taxi, grocery store, or elevator or something. (Yet another reason to have prepared for natural childbirth.) Sometimes it just happens. Visualize exactly what you don't want to happen so that no matter what happens, you'll feel prepared, and you'll know you can handle it. Birth just does its own thing – every time!

Meditation and visualization are incredibly powerful tools to manifest anything we want in life. Every pregnant woman wants an easy labor and delivery, and a healthy, happy newborn. Visualize it, create it, and know that it's done.

Affirmations

If you already know about and use affirmations, I want to remind you to use them during your pregnancy. If you don't know what they are, listen up. Affirmations are sentences we say to ourselves over and over until they seep into our subconscious and become what we believe. They are the single best way I know of to create change in yourself.

Affirmations work best in the first person, the present tense, and in the positive. You can use my suggestions, or tailor them to your personal needs.

Some examples follow. Pick the one you need first, say it over and over until it feels real, then move on to another. Writing them over and over is effective too.

- I am perfectly capable of birthing.

- My pregnancy and birth are perfect just the way they are.

- I am strong.

- I am happy.

- Pregnancy is natural, normal, healthy, and safe for me and my baby.

- I am calm and relaxed.

- I am beautiful and wondrous.

- My baby and I are safe.

- Labor and birth are totally normal, natural and safe.

Know thyself. Those were the only two words inscribed on the Greek Temple at Delphi circa 1100 BC. Write down the affirmations you need to change *your perception* of yourself and the world around you. Then make them your mantra.

Part II

Preparing
for
Baby

- Chapter 14 -
Becoming a Mother

No one ever really made it clear to me that motherhood would be the **single greatest experience of my life.**

The most poignant thing about motherhood for me is that everything I do now effects someone else *directly*. Every choice, every decision, every thought, every mood. I now must be the best student, joy-seeker, and conscious self-helper that I can be.

Now is all that matters.

Think For Yourself

If you haven't already begun to think for yourself, now is the time. No one knows what you should do for yourself or for your child better than you. No doctor, no relative, no book. Yes, you can ask sage and respected people their advice, and perhaps you will take it. Just remember that everyone is human, just like you. If something you hear or read doesn't resonate with you, listen to your inner guidance.

You also need to know who you are and what you believe. You are soon going to be charged with the task of guiding a new little being on the planet.

Your brain can only hold one thought at a time. All you have to do is keep that one thought a positive one, and you will be astounded at how wonderful your life becomes. Your magnet becomes a positive one. You attract love, opportunity, wealth, joy, friends, good books, the list goes on and on and on.

This power of positivity is something that's going to be so important to teach your child. We are all collectively creating this world we live in together. If you want your child to be happy, and you want the world to be a happy place, you need to get cracking. For more information on deliberate creation, listen to or read anything by Abraham-Hicks or Wayne Dyer.

Also, when it comes to thinking for yourself, you have to learn how to make good decisions. Every decision we make is either out of love or out of fear. If you stop and think about it, it's true. The only reason to say or do anything is out of love. When you're making a big decision, you can usually boil it down to whether it comes from love or fear. If you're making it out of fear, rethink your decision and make it out of love for yourself and/or out of love for another.

Pursue People and Decisions that Resonate

Things either resonate with you or they don't. By resonate, I mean harmonize. When two violins are in tune together and they're hanging on a wall, if you pluck one string on one violin, the same string on the violin next to it will vibrate. People are the same way. We vibrate, literally. Our cells are in vibration. When you get with someone with whom you resonate, you know it. It feels good. Birds of a feather flock together. When you hear music that you like, you know it. It resonates at a similar frequency as you.

Here on Earth, we people can actually consciously raise our vibrations. When you practice positive thinking, you will raise your vibration. You may not be able to hang with some of the same negative folks you used to enjoy. That's okay. In fact, I'd recommend dumping anyone with a negative vibration, because you'll just start resonating with it again. Once we reach adulthood, we have control over our environment – who's in it, what music is playing, what's on TV, where we live, what we eat.

Start creating your dream environment, not just for you, but also for the child inside you. For more on resonance, read Gary Zukav's *The Seat of the Soul*.

Become conscious of the people and things that resonate with you and follow your inner guidance. Life is wonderful, magical and beautiful, and it needs to be.

You're about to have a baby.

- Chapter 15 -
It All Starts Before You Are Born

Your child is exposed to everything you are. This is especially true for the things you hear and feel. Well, and of course, the things you eat, drink, breathe and inject.

There is an amazing book called *The Secret Life of the Unborn Child* by Thomas Verny. He goes into detail about studies that have been done on pregnant women who have struggled with various issues. For instance, there was a study done on the children of women whose husbands were at war during their pregnancies. Just imagine for a moment how anxious you would be if your husband/ partner were at war. The child inside you is connected to you in every way – physically, emotionally, hormonally, psychically etc. The children born to women under these circumstances were 100 times more likely than other children to have physical and emotional disturbances as adults.

What we've learned from this is that women have an enormous ability to shape their children's personalities while they are pregnant. "Her tools are her thoughts and feelings, and with them she has the opportunity to create a human being favored with more advantages than previously thought possible."[17]

If you are optimistic and happy, your child will be hard-wired to be the same way. If you are negative and worried all of the time, ditto for your kid.

Fetuses hear everything. It might be muffled, but they hear it nonetheless. They hear happy singing, beautiful music, and the lilt of various languages. They also hear discord and arguing.

They **feel meaning** rather than actually understanding it. They know if they are wanted or unwanted. In other words, your self-esteem starts before you're born.

Even if you don't want your child, you'd better start pretending you do, mainly to start believing you do, because your child's going to know if you're pretending. *Wanted children are advantaged even before birth.*

Teach Your Child Now

Another fascinating reality is that since your child can really hear you while he is inside you, you can actually make him "smarter" by being aware of this. If you talk to your child every day the way you would talk to a baby, using real vocabulary words, singing the ABC's, and counting, he will learn these things at an incredible rate of speed once he's out here in the world. Speak to him in your second language. Use big words. Talk about God or whatever you call It. Listen to beautiful music. Tell your baby you love him.

And then, when he's born, do the same thing. Never talk baby talk. Babies are innately more intelligent than we are because they are the next generation; they are more evolved than we.

Read baby books to them and start teaching them nouns from the get go. Language and intelligence build each other. If you've been pointing out the ceiling fan, the dog, etc., your child's language will develop as quickly as it can, and that's fun for everybody.

There is another wonderful book called *How to Have a Smarter Baby* by Susan Ludington-Hoe. I started reading this book when my baby was around four months old, but the book recommended starting before the child is born. Oops. I want my children to have the best life possible, and what I know is that it starts while you are pregnant.

If you are a happy and positive woman, chances are that you'll have a happy and positive baby. If you're not a happy and positive woman, I'm suggesting that you become one in order to give your child a fighting chance.

- Chapter 16 -
Things to Procure While You Are Pregnant

There is so much to choose from these days when it comes to baby products that it's really hard to know which products are going to really suit you the best. So, here's my list of the things I was really glad I found:

- Cloth diapers etc. if you're going to go that route

- Birth announcements

- A pop-out car seat

- Clothes

- A crib

- A changing table

- An infant bathtub

- A boppy pillow if you intend to nurse

- Your birth kit (if you're having a home birth)

- Non-toxic (in other words, not plastic) baby bottles

- A blender or baby food grinder

- A 2-4 week supply of food for your whole family

- Baby (and Earth) friendly detergent

- Weleda baby cream and diaper rash cream

- A sling and/or Baby Bjorn

- A video camera

- Bouncy Seat – Fisher Price Flutter & Chime Calming

- Vibrations

- Neglectomatic

- . . . and there's more.

But first, just let me state a hindsight opinion. I wish I had been more conscious when it came to my baby registries. I just followed the other lemmings over to Target and Babies "R" Us. I didn't set a good example for my friends or turn my mom's friends on to organic possibilities. I probably helped the Chinese economy a little, and I ended up with a bunch of plastic stuff that's probably still out-gassing in my baby's nursery.

Obviously, shopping locally helps your economy. If you can find some local mom and pop shops that have some dreamy items like organic cotton baby clothes, organic baby wash, Weleda baby products, wooden toys, and cloth diapers, set up a registry with them. It would be worth the bit of extra time. The other way to go is to find a couple of websites that you like. There are many of them, but they tend to come and go, so just Google "natural baby products" and set up a registry with one or two.

There are usually a few things that we can't do without that seem to need to come from Target or Walmart. I'm referring to things like strollers, boppy pillows, highchairs, car seats, etc. If you're really opposed to shopping at these places, you usually can find gently used items at your local children's reseller.

The List:

Cloth Diapers, etc.

I'll go into great detail later, but as a quick reference, you'll need about 2 dozen newborn Chinese prefold diapers, 3-4 dozen regular size, 6 newborn size Bummies brand diaper covers, and about 12 smalls. You'll need a diaper pail with a washable liner, and about 40 cloth wipes. I spent about $400 at first, and then another $200 on miscellaneous items over the next two years, including a dozen cotton, washable training pants. Over these two years, it has saved us thousands.

Birth Announcements

This one is really cool. Most people you know are going to want to know your baby was born (all the details with a picture too) before she goes off to college. Seriously, it's just nice to announce the birth in proximity to the birth. However, the very last things you're going to want to make time for during the first week of your baby's life are announcement shopping and addressing envelopes. Here is a really cool tip that I was given, used, and will most definitely pass along.

Go ahead and get the announcements ready a month before your due date (all but the photo, of course). I bought blank cards and designed my own on my computer, just leaving out the date, baby name, weight, length etc. I addressed and stamped the envelopes. Within two weeks of the birth, I had sent away for photos on line and received them. All I had to do was open the document, add the missing pieces, print, and stuff . . . which is still a lot to do, but I could do most of that lying in my bed with my newborn.

Pop-Out Car Seat

When I was feeling rushed and overwhelmed during my registration experience at Target, I picked out what turned out to be a great toddler car seat. It seemed like the thing to get because it would last from newborn to 40 pounds. The problem didn't arise until I finally started taking my baby out of the house after he was a month old.

Newborns fall asleep all the time, and when they do, you want them to stay that way. If you're running to the grocery store and your little angel falls asleep in the car, uh-oh, you have to wake them up and put them in the sling. And you don't want to do that. On our second outing, we stopped by Babies "R" Us and just forked over the $130 for the Graco infant car seat that pops out into a carrier. This product rocked my world for almost a year. Even if my sweetie was awake, I could just pop the thing out and fit it right into the grocery cart facing me. We could pop him out and take him into a restaurant with ease. I don't know how I missed the necessity of this product before giving birth, but I did. Perhaps so you won't.

You are also going to want the non-pop-out car seat as well. The infant one that you can pop out only fits little babies. At age two, we're still using the one from our registry. Register for both.

One more thing worth mentioning is the infant car-seat insert. This is a great, inexpensive item that keeps the little baby's head snug while she is still too small for the car seat. You can also roll up some cloth on either side of the baby's head to keep it from falling to the side.

Babies' heads tend to fall forward in the car seat when they sleep. My husband and I couldn't agree on whether or not we should constantly be messing with the baby's head. I did a little research on the web, and I found only one incidence of a baby dying in this way; however, he was left in the car that way for hours. It doesn't look very comfortable, so we always tried to fix it. You'll see. And since your baby faces backwards for a long time, it's nice to get a mirror that attaches to the headrests in the back seat, so you can glance in the rearview mirror and see how your baby is doing.

Baby Clothes (Don't really get them yet)

You really don't need many, and people are going to give you a ton. If you don't know the sex of your baby, just get a few packages of white onesies (which you can tie-dye later). Something else to keep in mind is that you don't know what size your baby is going to be when he is born. Premies actually have their own size – super, extra tiny. My friend, Andrea, gave birth to a thirteen-pound bouncing baby girl who was already in 6-9 month sizes at birth. Everything she bought for 0-3 months and 3-6 months was useless to her.

Unless you've done this before, you have no idea how fast babies grow that first year. They're out of sizes way before you think they'll be. Once the baby's here, you can go to the local resale shop and buy 4 times as many clothes as you could afford new. When they're on to the next size and grandma keeps sending new clothes, you'll be glad you didn't spend a fortune on baby clothes.

Crib

This is a no-brainer unless you're doing the co-sleeping thing. We tried the family bed, but ended up using the crib. One thing to keep in mind when buying a crib is the distance between the bars. All cribs manufactured these days adhere to strict rules so that babies can't get their little heads stuck between the bars. If you're like me and prefer antiques, just make sure that it's not one of the really old ones where the bars are far apart. My mom assures me that none of her children died this way, but I'm under the impression that this has happened once or twice, and there's nothing pleasant about that.

The other thing to keep in mind is to get a nice firm mattress. Babies are just like little adults. They do better on a firm mattress, but not a brick. A rule of thumb when picking out a mattress – your child will probably like what you like.

Changing Table

I thought that this cute little table we had would work fine. And it did, until like six months and 1800 diaper changes later, when I realized that the "changing" table had been just a little too short for me all that time. Your changing table needs to be a very comfortable height for you. If you're bending over a little too far every time you put her down and pick her up, your back will be screaming at you in a few months.

I still cheaped out and instead of buying a proper table at this point, I started doing spread-legged partial squats with a straight back. It's called body mechanics for diaper changing. I do the same thing when my back's hurting and I have to wash dishes. Yeah – sexy . . .

Infant Bathtub

Babies are slippery when wet and they don't really "fit" in the sink. This is a relatively cheap item that makes bath time a breeze. It's a plastic little tub with a spongy insert that fits nicely on top of the sink. You can use your little sprayer, get baby good and clean, and you can stand up the whole time. It also travels to Grandma's pretty well.

A "Boppy" Pillow

If you intend to nurse, this thing saves your arms. And as a bonus, when your baby starts to do "tummy time," it's a great prop to put under him on the floor. You can also kind of prop baby up in it as a little seat for a while. This is just a very mommy friendly product. In fact, my friend, Rachel, has two Boppy pillows that she has kept just for when nursing friends come over. Suffice it to say Rachel is so thoughtful of others, that she might as well be a professional friend. While you're making your wish list, put one of these down too – a professional friend with two Boppy pillows, 4000 children's books, great taste in children's music, and contagious patience.

Your Birth Kit (for home birth)

Your midwife will explain this for you in greater detail. The birth kit includes all of the disposable and one-use things that you will need at the time of your birth, like postpartum underwear, pads, the little suction thingy called a DeLee they use to clear the baby's breathing passages after birth, disposable under pads, sterile gloves, sterile lubricating jelly, sterile povidone scrub brush, sterile gauze pads, alcohol preps, and more. It also includes things that the midwives will leave with you after the birth like the little knit newborn hats, a digital thermometer, and the ever-important bulb syringe. (You'll use this thing to get boogers out for years.) Don't put off getting your birth kit if you're having a home birth. If you're doing it in the hospital, there is no need.

Non-toxic Baby Bottles

This was something I found out about way too late and sure wish I had known. Look into glass bottles, especially if you're planning to microwave or use a bottle warmer. It's been found that when we heat things in plastic, the plastic leaches out into whatever it is that we're about to consume. And you think, "Glass? What if it breaks?" Well, I thought that too. The bottle won't break if you or some other adult is holding it while the baby nurses. Popular thought today is that it's a no-no to prop baby up with a bottle. Best thing is the boob, but if you're doing a bottle, hold the baby while you do it, so that at least he gets the holding, loving, and warmth of human touch.

Blender or Baby Food Grinder

I was told to get the little hand held baby food grinder, so I did. If you have or can get a blender, just skip the little grinder. It's great if you don't have anything else, but if you have a blender, the grinder is a useless pain in the @#$, and the blender makes a much better texture.

2-4 week supply of food for your whole family

If you're using a midwife, she will make it clear to you that you need to stay in bed for a minimum of 2 weeks after the birth, so having food stocked up is a must. Get all of the staples – soups, pastas, frozen goodies, and anything that your partner feels comfortable cooking because you my dear, will need to be in bed with your baby. If any friends or family offer to bring you meals during that time, take them up on it! Fresh food is always the most nutritious, so hopefully your partner or a friend will be able to swing by the market and get some fresh fruits and veggies during this, the best month of your life.

Baby/Earth Friendly Detergent

My favorite is Seventh Generation Baby Laundry Detergent. I used it from diapers through training pants. Baby's skin is often too sensitive for the chemicals found in conventional detergents. Always wash new clothes before putting them on your child. Whenever we washed clothes or diapers at someone else's house, my baby would get a little red skin rash. I learned, and started traveling with good detergent, shampoo, soap, etc. If you simply have to wash clothes or diapers with conventional detergent, just be sure to rinse twice.

Weleda Baby Cream and Diaper Rash Cream

The skin of a newborn was not what I expected. It's only been exposed to air since birth, and after a week or two it starts to peel. Weleda baby cream is an amazing natural skin softener meant just for babies. Get 2 or 3 tubes of it. Apply it generously to your newborn's entire body every day for weeks. You both will love it. Also, I never found an all-natural diaper cream that worked better than the Weleda brand. It's a little more expensive, but you'll end up just throwing the others away anyway.

Sling, Moby Wrap and/or Baby Bjorn

I had all three and loved all three. Baby wearing is best for everyone. Babies feel so secure up against us. The Moby Wrap is awesome for the newborn stage, and the Bjorn isn't. Wait a few months to put your baby in the Bjorn. There's a school of thought out there that it's not a good idea to prop up a baby's head until he can do so himself. If his neck muscles aren't strong enough to do it himself, then his neck probably can't handle it. My husband was quite partial to the Baby Bjorn because it's very easy to put on. The Moby is more comfortable, but a hassle to don.

A Video Camera

If you don't already have one, you really ought to spring for it. Not only will you enjoy watching your child's first years, but she will appreciate it in years to come.

Flutter & Chime Calming Vibrations

This little bouncy seat was given me by my sister-in-law who had twins and two of these rockin' little seats. She found that she could feed them both at the same time while bouncing them and keeping them happy. We've just loved the portability of the thing. I'd have one in every room if I had the money. It's a step up from just laying the baby on the floor for a while. You definitely need to lay your baby on the floor when you can so that it she learns to roll and creep; however, sometimes it's nice for baby to be propped up a little so she can see what you're doing. My babies love sitting in this thing while I cook or clean. To me, this is indispensable, and I wouldn't have even known about it if it hadn't been given to me. Thanks, Ange.

The "Neglectomatic"

That's the name we have given the freestanding battery powered swing/seat that we move around the house. It's a little cumbersome to move, and it eats up "D" batteries, but it's another spot for baby when your arms and back give up. This is not a "must have" like the bouncy seat mentioned above, but it is definitely worth mentioning as a luxury.

The following are things I'm really glad we had, but you don't necessarily need them before you have the baby:

Bibs

I received a gift of seven little tiny terry cloth bibs and wondered what in the world I would need them for. Each one had a different day of the week embroidered on it. When my first son was about 4 months old and starting to teethe, he also started to drool, and he didn't stop for about 4 more months. He was, at every moment, like a Great Dane in August. He would soak the little fronts of his shirts over and over. Finally, after I had changed his clothes three times one day I remembered those little bibs. I ended up buying seven more. He wore a bib as part of his outfit for months, and I was so grateful for those little things.

The other bib that I found (and still find) to be indispensable is a firm plastic coated canvas one that folds up and snaps to make a little crumb catcher in front. I have two of them that we have used for two years. The brand I adore is Dex Products. Every time a parent from a former generation sees my kids in this bib they say, "Boy, I wish we had had those."

Cloth Grocery Cart Cover

This is quite a luxury when shopping. Babies tend to put their mouths right on the handle of the shopping cart. Buy one of these cart covers, and your worries are over.

"First Years" Swing Arm Booster Seat

It is the only one we've needed so far, and my son is two and a half. It's easy to clean, it's portable, it's safe, and just goes on one of the chairs at your table. The best thing about it is the "captivity" element. My son sits at the table and eats with us at every meal. He is the only two-year-old I know that does this. I attribute it 100% to this miraculous booster seat.

- Chapter 17 -
Breastfeeding

Thank heavens we're figuring this out again as liberated women. There is no substitute for what took millions of years to evolve as the perfect nutritive substance for baby humans. Breast milk nourishes us in every way. In fact, it's all we need in the way of nutrition for the first six months of life.

We simply have to relearn how to do it. Most of our mothers can't help us. In fact, my mom never learned how to breast feed properly and thought her milk really wasn't good enough. She thought she "dried up" after four months with my sister. I'm really impressed that in the 1960's she was even trying at all.

There are a few reasons why I know that my mom wasn't breastfeeding properly. The most obvious is that breast milk doesn't typically "dry up." On the contrary, it gets more and more established until the day comes that you start to wean. Even then you can't get it to stop producing. A month after my baby was entirely weaned, I could still squeeze milk out of my nipple. If I had needed to start breastfeeding again at that point, the faucets would have been happy to be turned on. There is even an article in Mothering Magazine (Jan/Feb 2001) written by an adoptive mother who managed to produce milk for her baby just by pumping and nursing until her breasts responded.[18] There's also a book out there called *Breastfeeding the Adopted Baby* by Debra Stewart Peterson.

Something else that has come to my attention lately is called the "breast crawl." The truth is that human babies, in the first moments of life, if they are placed on the mother's chest between her breasts, have the strength and instinct not only to find the breast, but to make a primitive "crawl" to it and latch on with no help. Look up YouTube videos for proof. Human babies, like all other mammals were designed to nurse, instinctually.

I'm pretty certain that what happened to my mom is what happens to most women when left to their own devices to figure out breastfeeding. They simply don't shove enough nipple into the baby's mouth, and they don't nurse often enough. We think our nipples are the little pencil eraser ends, but that's not the part that produces milk. When you're nursing properly, the entire areola is being sucked. It's by pressing down and squeezing the milk ducts way back from the nipple that the milk comes shooting out.

How to Breastfeed

- Shove all of the areola into the little tiny newborn's mouth. It will not gag. It really takes three hands to do it until you both get the hang of it, so get your partner to help. One hand squeezes the areola and shoves it way in. One hand holds the baby's head tipped way back. One hand opens the baby's mouth really wide. Side-lying position is easiest and most comfortable. Lie on your side with your arm out of the way. Put a pillow behind your back. Skin to skin contact is very important. Pull the baby way up next to your body and make sure that her little head is looking UP to your breast. Head back, mouth open, whole nipple in.

- Bite a bullet every two hours for the next month. Seriously, the first thirty seconds of nursing after the baby latches on hurts like a mother, but in about a month, you will be entirely numb.

- For the first two weeks, use side-lying position (you need to be horizontal for your uterus to heal) and massage the entire breast toward the nipple occasionally to make sure that all of the ducts are emptied. After the first two weeks, you can change the baby's position every time you breast feed. At night you'll likely want to do side-lying position, so during the day try football hold, classic Madonna, and any other weird 12 o'clock, 2 o'clock, 9 o'clock position with pillows that you can figure out. This ensures that all of your milk ducts are getting emptied and you are less apt to end up with a clogged duct and potential infection. After a while you can just go back to massaging the breast now and then if you don't want to do a bunch of holds.

- Put Lansinoh cream on your nipples in between nursings for the first couple of weeks. It keeps your nipples from getting dry and cracked.

- Try to start nursing on alternating breasts each time you nurse. Early nursing can last up to 30 minutes a breast, but you'll soon be switching after 10 minutes. If you can't remember which breast you started with (believe me, it happens!) you can put a safety pin in the side of your bra where you start.

- Have a glass of water beside you while you nurse. Nursing makes you thirsty.

Those First Weeks of Nursing

Breastfeed every time your newborn cries no matter what anyone else says. The first few days, they're only getting colostrum, and I shouldn't say only, because this is one of the most important boosts your immune system ever gets, but what they want is milk. They are unimaginably hungry. Every time you feed them, the closer your milk is to coming in and relieving you both.

When your baby latches on, it does hurt, but your nipples should never be raw or bloody. If they are, your baby is probably trying to nurse on the ends of your nipples. Try to push more of your breast into their mouth. During the first 2-4 weeks, even though the first minute of nursing is rather painful for the mother, do it as often as possible anyway. You're establishing your milk supply. If you nurse every 1-2 hours during the day, your baby might start sleeping through the night by 3-4 months old because they are getting enough calories during the day.

Wear a snug nursing bra for the first two weeks, 24 hours a day. It helps keep you from getting engorged, which is almost inevitable and very painful. Hot showers and cold cabbage leaves help with relief. Place the cold, preferably purple cabbage leaves directly inside your bra and replace as necessary. Wearing the nursing bra will also hopefully help keep your boobs from sagging too much later in life.

Pumping

Pumping can relieve engorgement, but it also encourages more milk production, so it's a double-edged sword. I do, however, highly recommend pumping after engorgement is over. Pump and freeze for when Daddy or Grandma want to give a bottle or for when you go out to dinner and leave it for the babysitter. Be warned: about half way through dinner, your boobs will ache to be nursed and you'll wish you were home. My fat little baby never once even tasted "formula."

Pump and freeze so you can donate milk to the local milk bank. They take donations, and then they pasteurize the milk to be prescribed to preemies in the hospital. Your breast milk is like gold.

There is something worth mentioning called "nipple confusion." It sounds like a band name, but it's an actual phenomenon that occurs when a baby who is given a pacifier or a bottle too early forgets how to nurse on the breast. The sucking method is different. My son never took to a pacifier, although we did offer it, and we waited to give him some breast milk from a bottle until he was several months old. Nipple confusion was never an issue for us, but I'm glad it was on my radar.

Benefits of Breastfeeding

Breastfeeding is so easy, so natural, and free. There are no bottles to wash or heat. Mom's milk is warm and ready whenever your baby needs it. It's a natural sleeping aid, and I always called it the "magic elixir," which came in quite handy when my baby was learning to crawl and walk. Every time he crashed and cried, there was the boob to make it all better. We nursed taking off and landing in airplanes to relieve the pressure on his ears. God knows I wish every mother on an airplane could figure this one out.

It's unbelievable to me that so many women either think they can't nurse or simply opt to pay oodles of money for a "formula" created in a laboratory somewhere. After they buy the stuff, they then have to get up 3 or 4 times a night and heat it while their baby is crying and waiting. While my baby was still feeding at night, he'd wake up and let me know it was time. I'd lie down beside him and usually sleep while he nursed. When a woman nurses her baby, a wonderful relaxing hormone called prolactin is released into her system. It's like a chill pill every time we nurse.

When we deprive our children of our milk, we just can't be certain of all we're depriving them. The immunity of the mother is certain, as we know that this gets passed on through breast milk. My child had three minor colds during the first 2 years of his life. I've heard averages between 8 and 12 illnesses a year are the norm for babies in America. Breast milk passes along hormones, antibodies, omega fatty acids, and intestinal flora; these are things that might deter illness for a lifetime.

Also, the benefits to the mother are enormous. During the first few days after birth, nursing releases hormones that contract the uterus and reduce postpartum bleeding. Long-term nursing lowers a woman's risk of breast, ovarian, and endometrial cancers, and reduces her risk of osteoporosis and bone fracture as well.[19] Nursing babies also help their mothers to lose the "baby weight" by requiring lots of fat in the milk. They literally suck the fat right off of you, assuming you're not consuming loads of fat in your diet. If you continue eating a healthy diet, you'll love the way nursing helps you to get back to your pre-pregnancy weight.

How Long?

As far as how long you should nurse goes, only you will know the answer to that. All I know for sure is the longer, the better. The health benefits of nursing are cumulative for the child, from colostrum the first few days that set up flora in the intestines, to after six weeks, lowering rates of many diseases. Long-term nursing (more than a year) protects against diabetes, asthma, childhood cancers, and obesity, just to name a few. It also enhances neurological development that may result in higher IQ's and better eyesight.[20]

I originally planned to nurse my first son for 6 months, but when 6 months rolled around, there was no need to stop. I eventually weaned when he was 2, but some moms keep it up until their children are 3 and 4, which is par for the course in many developing countries. In other words, long-term nursing is normal for the human species.

Seek Out Help

My experience leads me to say that chances are you're going to need someone knowledgeable to help you get your baby to latch on the first few times. If you're delivering at home with a midwife, you're covered. If you're delivering in the hospital, make sure they know that you'll burn the place down if anyone gives your baby formula without your consent, and then see if they have a lactation consultant available. Otherwise, have a doula at your birth or get books on the subject from your local library and find your local chapter of La Leche League. They will help you with every aspect of one of the most amazing experiences you'll ever have as a mom, breastfeeding.

It is true that now and then a mother and baby for some reason cannot nurse. Some babies really do bite. Some nipples really can't be latched on to. Don't feel bad if you try and try, but it doesn't work. You tried. They used to have wet nurses for this. Now they have formula. But before you give up, find someone knowledgeable (lactation consultant, midwife, doula, La Leche League member, or even a friend who has recently breast-fed a newborn) to make sure that you really can't nurse.

I'd like to reiterate that if at first you don't succeed, you try, try again. And if you still don't succeed, don't sweat it. It's not the end of the world. You're not a failure. You're the formula goddess. Love it.

- Chapter 18 -
Cloth Diapers

Yep, duped by our own beautiful creation, Capitalism.

Here's what I'd been led to believe prior to the birth of my son: cloth diapers are a total pain, a throwback to pioneer women doing loads of laundry and packing heat at the same time. I saw diaper pins and bloody fingers. I saw diaper blowouts everywhere, leaking all over God's creation. I saw reeking, poopy hampers begging to be put off another day. I knew that disposable diapers were filling up our landfills, but the aforementioned images were ingrained.

How unbelievably misinformed I was. Even after deciding to use cloth diapers, I bought a package of every single size of disposable diaper there was, simply being certain that I'd need one from time to time. We never did.

A few months prior to the birth, we were told that a diaper service would make it all okay. We bought 5 dozen cloth diapers, a dozen diaper covers, a diaper pail and pail liner, and 40 cloth wipes for a total of about $400.

We called to set up the diaper service, and you can imagine how bummed we were to find out that they didn't deliver out as far as our house. We were all on our own. But like I say, everything's always perfect. If it hadn't turned out that way, I wouldn't be able to tell you that we've been duped – even the part about needing a diaper service.

For the first month after our son was born, my husband washed all of the diapers while I was joyfully held captive in my big bed by my baby and my healing uterus. I thought he was being so heroic as he never complained once. As soon as I took over the diaper washing, I realized that there was nothing to complain about. And I am not exaggerating in the least. I cannot figure out why Americans have gotten so hooked on disposable diapers. And I'm the first person on Earth to appreciate something that really does make life easier. I love hot, running water, computers, the Internet, air travel, and the list goes on and on. On my list of things that make life better: cloth diapers.

And don't let your mother or grandmother convince you otherwise; cloth diapering has come a long way, baby. The diaper wraps they make these days are user-friendly thanks to Velcro and snaps, and they almost never leak. The one time that my son had a really gnarly blowout, I'm sure it would have blown out of anything, cloth or disposable.

The first 2-3 weeks, you won't use wraps at all because your baby will just be too tiny to wear them, so you'll have to struggle with diaper pins until the wrap just neatly velcros or snaps it all together.

What to Buy

I already listed most of what you need to get your cloth diapering going, but here goes a real, vertical list.

- 2-3 dozen newborn size Chinese prefolds

- 3-4 dozen regular size Chinese prefolds

- 6 newborn size Bummis diaper wraps

- 8-12 small size Bummis diaper wraps (if you have a preemie or a large baby, adjust the sizes)

- 30-40 cloth wipes

- a 5 gallon diaper pail

- a 5 gallon diaper pail liner

- a small "dry bag" to put dirties in when you're out with the diaper bag

- some organic liquid baby wash

- * a very gentle detergent

- about 10 cloth (hemp or cotton) diaper inserts

What to Do

Here's what you do. When there's a pee pee diaper, it goes directly into the pail. When there's a poopy one, you drop it in the toilet. The same goes for the poopy diaper wraps. You come back in a few minutes and squeeze it out. I know that sounds gross, but it's really not gross until your baby starts eating solid food, and by then you're used to it. I know my toilet is clean, and I know what goes into my baby. If you don't like this idea, just have a "wet" bucket, a bucket with water in it that you drop the diapers into. Squeeze them out at the end of the day and add them to the pail.

You can use rubber gloves if you want to. This is what I did when I was visiting relatives. If you really can't fathom the idea of touching poo, they make contraptions that squeeze the diapers for you.

But let me go ahead and warn you, you can't be a parent and not touch poo or pee or vomit or snot. The day will come. You *will* catch vomit bare-handed and you really won't mind that much. Or at least you'll get over it.

When you get close to needing more clean diapers, you dump the pail into the washing machine. Do one rinse cycle with cold water. Then do one hot water wash with a teeny amount of gentle detergent. Make sure that the diapers have plenty of room to agitate in the wash. You will be amazed at how sudsy the water gets. You will never need bleach. There is no need. Our rivers, lakes and marine life will thank you, too. If your diapers get a little poop stained, just hang them to dry from time to time in the bright sun. It's amazing how it bleaches the diapers. There's no need for fabric softener either.

We never ran out of diapers and had to run to the store. We only had to wash about twice a week. No biggie. You don't even have to fold them, just stack them.

Cloth Wipes

I also love the cloth wipes. They look like thick, small washcloths with super reinforced stitching around the entire edge so that they withstand 2000 washes.

Here's what you do, and this seriously takes 30 seconds each morning:

- Take 6 or so cotton wipes, more at first, less after a while

- Put some water with a little dab of baby wash in a bowl, stir, add the dry wipes

- Soak up the solution and squeeze them out.

- Put them in a ziplock bag and you have all natural, reusable wipes.

- Just throw them in the diaper pail and wash with the diapers. Environment and baby booty approved.

Considerations

Diaper Rash?

Diaper rash can occur in any type of diaper and requires immediate attention. In seventeen months of cloth diapering, my son had only two minor bouts with it. If we ever saw a little pink on his bottom, we put cream on right away or let him go diaperless for a while. Diaper rash really wasn't on our radar very much, and I attribute this to cloth diapers and the frequency with which we changed them.

Diaper Service?

Since we started using cloth diapers, I understand that using a diaper service isn't all that much better environmentally speaking, than using the disposables. Diaper services have to wash 3 times and use bleach because they are putting everybody's fecal matter together to wash. Using a diaper service is better than going with disposables, but if you really want to be environmentally friendly, wash your diapers yourself.

Disposable Diapers?

Studies have recently shown that disposable diapers increase scrotal temperatures in boys to the point of causing low sperm counts as adults. Researchers have also found that when mice are exposed to clean disposables, they have a higher incidence of asthma.[21]

The other argument against disposables is that whatever that chemical wonder gel is that soaks up pee to where you can't even feel it, it's sitting up cozy against your baby's genitals for years. Considering that we're finding chemicals in our baby's blood at a truly alarming rate,[22] I'll take organic cotton that I wash myself, thank you.

All-in-Ones?

All-in-ones are convenient, but not necessary. I bought a few just to try them out. Basically, they are the cloth diaper and the wrap all in one. When you use real wraps, if the diaper gets wet only, you can reuse the wrap until it gets poop on it. The all-in-ones are only good for one change, even if it's just pee, and they're really expensive. Next time, I'd just use the prefolds and wraps.

You're also going to want some "inserts" for when your baby starts peeing more abundantly and for nighttime.

Large-Wraps?

I never needed the "large" size wraps or diapers because I don't believe in keeping toddlers in diapers. I love the Bummis brand training pants, though.

- Chapter 19 -
Circumcision

I would say that this is a decision only you can make for your son, but that would be far from true. It's a decision that your son can make for himself as well.

Aside from Jews and Muslims who practice circumcision for religious purposes, people are starting to realize that there's no reason whatsoever to have a baby boy circumcised. There have been cases where circumcisions were botched, and sparing you the gory details, little boys have been "sexually reassigned" as little "girls."[23] Circumcision is traumatic genital mutilation that is extremely painful. In a modern country where most people have access to baths everyday, it's an archaic ritual that serves no purpose.

The American Academy of Pediatrics proclaims that the "data isn't sufficient to recommend routine neonatal circumcision."[24] People are catching on, but we still need to get the word out.

There is a wonderful group of doctors out there called Doctors Opposing Circumcision (D.O.C.). Part of their mission statement says, "These doctors recognize that no one has the right to forcibly remove sexual body parts from another individual. They also believe that "doctors should have no role in this painful, unnecessary procedure inflicted on the newborn."[25]

My father, the conservative, quiet, southern, retired attorney, has never said much about his private life ever. He's a man of few, yet very effective words. Nevertheless, I remember him saying several times during my life that when it comes to circumcision, he wishes that someone had simply given him the choice. If he had wanted to be circumcised, it could have been a decision he made for himself. So, I suppose I've always known that if I had a little boy, I would never allow anyone to unnecessarily take a knife to his little body. I could never do it.

I may be simply pointing out a trend because most of the little boys I know these days aren't circumcised. In fact, the national circumcision rate was down to 56% in 2006 (from a high of 85% in 1965) according to the Circumcision Reference Library.[26]

Even at 56%, we're still the most pathetic in the world when it comes to non-religious, medically unnecessary, neonatal circumcision. Non-English speaking countries have rates near 0%, and of other English speaking countries, Australia has the highest incident at 13%. (England is at 2.1 %)[27]

Coax the Foreskin back?

So, if you end up choosing to save that little foreskin and thus the sensitivity of the natural head of the penis, something you don't know that will become a controversy, is whether or not you should very gently help the foreskin to loosen up and pull back. There are very differing opinions out there on this one, and the jury's still out. We need to talk to young men whose mothers practiced both schools of thought and see who's got the most trouble-free foreskin.

One school says that for the first two years of life, a couple times a week during a diaper change or bath, GENTLY coax the foreskin back ever so slightly. It shouldn't necessarily retract for years, but you're encouraging it to do so, and you're teaching the boy to clean down there from a young age.

Also, in newborns there occurs something called smegma, which is basically a combination of skin cells, oils, and moisture, which appears as a cheese-like substance between the head of the penis and the foreskin. It can even run down the length of the shaft of the penis. It is nothing to worry about, but you can gently coax some of it out if you want to when you are doing the gentle foreskin stretch.

There is a big difference in gently coaxing and really pulling back the foreskin. *Never let anyone pull back the foreskin!* This includes your doctor. It is very painful and can even require emergency surgery.

The other school of foreskin thought is to do nothing. The foreskin will retract on its own by the time the boy needs it to, and a tight baby foreskin is helping to keep the fecal matter in the diaper away from the glans (head of the penis).

I have subscribed to the former coaxing method, and I've been very pleased with my son's foreskin experience. At age three, he has a perfect little package with a trouble-free foreskin.

Whichever school of thought you buy into, at least give yourself the choice and keep the foreskin. Do the research for yourself. A man can always get himself circumcised if he wants to. I know of one grown man who made this decision. He was a medical doctor, and I get the feeling he was anesthetized for the procedure.

- Chapter 20 -
Vaccinations

Whether or not to vaccinate has been a hot topic for several years now. Across the board, vaccinations have historically been a good thing. They have all but eradicated several hideous diseases from our world. A very small percentage of children have always had adverse reactions to vaccinations and still do. I recently found out that the three-year-old daughter of a friend of mine has had two occurrences of shingles because of the chicken pox vaccine they gave her!

My midwife believes in vaccinations. She believes in the world of good that they have done and continue to do. So I did my homework, but none too early. Since I had my baby at home, he wasn't subjected to the initial hepatitis shot that babies are routinely given in the hospital. He was also covered under my immunizations as long as I was breastfeeding him. I figured I'd give my son vaccinations, just not as many and not as close together as they recommend.

So, one day when my son was two months old, my husband was casually talking with his mom's cancer doctor and found out that the unbearably painful rash on his chest was shingles, not poison ivy as we had initially thought. Shingles are a reoccurrence of the chicken pox virus. The good oncologist thought it wise of us to get our baby a chicken pox shot, and as soon as possible.

I took my son immediately to the pediatrician for a chicken pox shot. At the $140 visit, I found out that they won't give a chicken pox shot to a baby that young and that it would be very difficult if not impossible for my baby to contract the disease, namely because

I was nursing him. That was a relief, but I still decided to get him the first round of vaccinations that they recommend so that I'd at least get my money's worth out of the visit.

At the time, I knew that there was some controversy around vaccinations, but I really wasn't sure what it was, so that night I started surfing the net to see what I could find about vaccinations. What I read weighed heavily upon me. I figured the controversy was around side effects, and yes, there is a small controversy about that, but the main one is over a side effect called autism.

I know autism all too well. I grew up next door to an autistic boy who was eventually institutionalized, and one of my best friends has a five-year-old daughter with autism. I've never seen anything cripple a family the way autism does.

If you don't already know someone affected by autism, you at least have heard of it. The latest jarring statistic is that 1 in 155 American children have autism. That statistic jumps to 1 in 100 for boys. No one is certain what is causing all of this autism. There could be a number of factors including genetic predisposition and environmental triggers.

However, there is debate going on about whether vaccines and the preservatives in them are a factor in the rise of autism. Two of the issues are the sheer number of shots a child is given at once, and the frequency with which they are given. The main vaccination in question is the MMR or measles/mumps/rubella shot. Hundreds of families swear that their toddler, who was talking normally at the time of the MMR vaccination, regressed within days of the vaccine to almost no words and slipped deep into the world of autism. It is difficult to prove. Because of this, the establishment doesn't want to cause panic over the practice of vaccination, and families who are dealing with autism want the whole world to know.

We have chosen to under-vaccinate our son. I refuse to give him the MMR vaccination until he's older. I have forms that I can sign and notarize and leave at any schools he attends that allow him exemption from vaccinations. It's that easy. In Texas, you don't have to vaccinate if you don't want to.

You simply write to:

Dept of State Health Services Immunization Branch

Mail Code 1946

PO Box 149347

Austin, TX 78714-9347

or

1100 W. 49th St.

Austin, TX 78756

Or fax: (512)458-7544

Phone: (512)458-7284

Call first to make sure nothing has changed.

You must ask in writing for the "Affidavit Exemption from Immunizations for Reasons of Conscience." Ask for the maximum number of forms you can receive, which is five. They will send you the exemption forms in the mail. In other states, you'll need to do your research.

When my son was two years old, my husband and I took him on a vacation to Central America. Again, we were inundated with caution for us all to get vaccines. So, I took my own advice. I researched it for myself. The CDC (Center for Disease Control) website is chock full of travel information. As far as the need for the MMR vaccine goes, in the areas where we were going, there had been no measles, and no rubella in the last 10 years. In 2006 there had been 140 cases reported of the mumps. With 1 in 100 boys in America having autism right now, I decided to chance the Central American mumps. We also opted to skip the family rounds of the hepatitis vaccine that had been recommended, and we didn't take antimalarial medication. We all came home unscathed.

~ ~ ~ ~ ~

Pertussis, or Whooping Cough has been going around lately, so I considered giving my four-month-old the vaccination. Ironically, my father had just sent me an article from Forbes magazine called "Get Vaccinated." So, once again, following my own advice, I started researching this topic yet again.

It's not just autism that has parents questioning the overuse of vaccinations these days. (Which, by the way, benefits pediatricians and drug companies, who in turn have the ability to press legislation) There are many children suffering from other issues like seizures, "staring spells," IQ loss, loss of muscular control, attention deficit, eye trouble (blindness, astigmatism, nystagmus), dyslexia, hearing loss, ear infections, athsma, migraines, and other physical disabilities, whose parents wonder if they were possibly caused by the pertussis vaccination.

The jury is still out on this one. The decision of whether or not to vaccinate is a tough one for parents because you're potentially endangering your child either way. The best advice I can give you is to do your homework, research the vaccination controversy to your heart's content, make the decision that works best for you, and then do it.

I highly recommend a book called *The Vaccine Book* by Dr. Sears. It is factually based and allows you to make your own decisions.

- Chapter 21 -
A Few Other Things to Consider

I am not a paranoid person at all. In fact, I'm far from it. But I am keenly aware that just because something is for sale doesn't necessarily make it safe. Back in high school in the late 1980's, people started talking about how aluminum was being linked to Alzheimer's disease. I was also aware that aluminum was the main ingredient in most deodorants. I've only used natural deodorant since. I still have never heard if putting aluminum daily on the really porous skin of the underarm has been proven as a cause for Alzheimer's, but I certainly don't want to be in the "variable" group of this mass experiment.

I know there could be a better system, but I have to trust that our government does the best it can to keep harmful products off the shelves. The problem is that sometimes we don't know a product is harmful until it's been used by millions of Americans for many years. The other problem is, and it's not really a problem, that we live in a free country. Sugar is probably one of the more harmful substances we consume, but if the USDA took it off the shelves, we'd have 100 million addicts freaking out about the fact that we're supposed to get to make our own decisions in this country. And we are. And we do.

That's why I've personally decided to monitor what goes into or touches my body, because I'm free to do so, and we have a wealth of choices in this amazing country. I don't have to wait for some study to be done in order to recognize intuitively that if pesticides kill pests, they're probably not something I want to eat. If you want a really good read about what you might consider not eating, check out *Skinny Bitch* by Rory Freedman and Kim Barnouin.

Things you might avoid:

It's worth noting that in a recent study on the umbilical cord blood of newborn infants, "researchers at two major laboratories found an average of 200 industrial chemicals and pollutants in umbilical cord blood from 10 babies born in August and September of 2004 in U.S. hospitals."[28]

Considering the myriad diagnoses of children these days for which the causes are unknown, here is a list of things that I personally have decided to avoid or minimize, especially during pregnancy and for my child. It is followed by a list of alternatives when possible.

- Anything treated with flame-retardants (especially pajamas) – try *untreated cotton*

- Plastic sippy cups and bottles – try *glass or stainless steel*

- Conventionally grown produce, meat, and poultry – try *organic*

- Disposable diapers, pull-ups and pads – try *cloth*

- Chemical cleaning products – try *natural cleaning products such as Vinegar, baking soda, lemon juice, tea tree oil etc.*

- Chemical pesticides and extermination – try *organic*

- Chemical fertilizers – try *compost and manure*

- Conventional make-up – try *Dr. Haushka's product line*

- Conventional perfume – try *essential oils*

- Cesarean Birth – try *only when necessary*

- T.V. – try *music, art, walking, playing, reading*

- Artificially colored or flavored food

- Vaccinations

- Ultrasounds (unnecessary ones)

- Conventional Pacifiers – try *natural rubber ones*

- Conventional detergents and dish soap

- Dryer sheets and fabric softener

- Conventional sunscreen

- New carpet

- Hand Sanitizer – try *soap and water*

- Anti-bacterial soap of all kinds (we really need bacteria)

- Conventional soap, shampoo, conditioner, shaving cream, lotions etc.

- Conventional toothpaste

Here is a list of the natural products, sometimes even organic, I have found that really are effective. I stand by each one of these products.

- Aubrey's "E Plus High C" deodorant. (It really works!)

- Dr. Haushka's cosmetic and facial cleansing line

- Ecover dishwasher powder (the cakes work the best)

- The entire line of Melaleuca products – laundry detergent, cleaning products

- Seventh Generation baby laundry soap

- Kiss My Face Moisture Shave (this product rocks)

Now, even if you avoid those unnecessary things really well and stick to the natural products as much as possible, you're still going to inhale, swallow, and rub up against your fair share just by being out in the world. That would be moderation, which is better than inundation. You'll stay in a hotel room with new carpet, eat antibiotic and hormone fed beef in a restaurant, see TV in the doctor's office, and end up with Halloween candy, but if you're avoiding them at home, then you and your baby should be cleaner than the next guy.

Part III

Tips on Getting
Pregnant
and
Staying That Way

- Chapter 22 -
Taking Charge of Your Fertility

This is a book title. *Taking Charge of Your Fertility*, by Toni Weschler could be required reading for women of child-bearing age.

It is so obvious when you're fertile, yet most of us don't know this. Toni makes it unquestionably clear. God bless you, Toni. You don't need to spend too many hormonally whacked years of your life taking the pill if you're avoiding pregnancy. You just need to know when *not* to have sex. Likewise, you don't need to spend emotionally disturbing months or years of your life getting fertility treatments on day 14 of your cycle in order to conceive when you typically ovulate on day 11 or 19.

The book also makes quite clear the need to chart your periods and temperatures. If you aren't doing this, you're not really trying that hard to get pregnant. You chart all three of the ovulation markers listed below. Over a few cycles you start to see your own patterns.

Three Ovulation Markers

There are three things our body does when ovulation kicks in. Two are recognizable in advance, and one is only recognizable in hindsight. As weird as it sounds the first time you hear it, cervical mucous is the key.

Mucous

You're looking for super stretchy, slippery mucous that looks like clear egg white. This is the "sperm highway." You are very fertile when you notice this type of mucous on your toilet paper or in your underwear. I never noticed it in my life until Toni called it to my attention. Now it seems that I was the only one who didn't know!

The easiest time to notice it is immediately following a bowel movement. Just reach a clean finger up against your labia and check out the quality of the discharge. Super stretchy and slippery . . . go getcha some. (Or, run like hell. It all depends on whether or not you want to be pregnant.)

The Placement and Feel of Your Cervix

Yes, another strange one. You actually have to reach up there and feel your cervix. As long as it's low and hard like the tip of your nose, you're not ovulating. As soon as it starts to move higher, open and soften, more like the feeling of your lips, you're about to ovulate.

Your Waking Temperature

The thing to watch for is a drop and then a spike in body temperature. Once you notice this however, you've usually just ovulated, but perhaps can still get pregnant. Over a few cycles you start to see how it works, and you can see the drop before the spike.

I can say from experience that charting is a hassle until you get used to it, and it's next to impossible if you are trying for child number two. You have to get in the habit of taking your temperature **every morning before your feet hit the floor.** As soon as you stand up, your temperature begins to rise, so you don't get an accurate temperature. If you have a baby that wakes up and wants you in the morning, you can't exactly tell him to wait while you take your temperature.

If you're not able to take your temperature daily before your feet hit the floor, but you want to know when you're about to ovulate, get some ovulation predictor kits at your local pharmacy. You have to be consistent and pee on the stick every day at approximately the same time of day. I've started as early as day 8 of my cycle, just to be sure that I haven't missed ovulation.

Toni's book has charts you can copy and use or a CD Rom so you can chart on your computer. She has you chart everything – sex, mood, feel of cervix, exercise, you name it. Over time, this becomes powerful information to have about yourself if you are trying to conceive.

Getting Pregnant

You want to have sex just before ovulation, and I've found that, for me, the stretchy mucous really arrives along side ovulation. **Your best bet is to have sex *everyday* around the time of ovulation.**

It's worth noting that many lubricants aren't sperm-friendly. There is one you can order online called "pre-seed" that has been formulated specifically to help you conceive. If you need a lubricant, I wouldn't use anything else.

My husband also took zinc along with his vitamins because it requires a lot of zinc to produce sperm. And I took a kelp supplement to make sure I was getting enough iodine to maintain a highly functioning thyroid. Those of us who like to use sea salt instead of iodized table salt don't usually get enough iodine, although I found iodized sea salt recently so this shouldn't be a problem any more.

Fertility Service Options You Can Do Yourself

If you're 35 or older, the consensus is that if you've tried to conceive for 6 months to no avail, it's time to start seeing a fertility specialist. I think this is hogwash. It took us 18 months to conceive both of my children, and one after I was 35. Big deal. I'm so glad that I trusted my instincts on this one. Instead of coughing up thousands and thousands of dollars just to be given chemistry-altering hormone treatments, invasive fertility treatments that can lead to octuplets, and months of heartache wondering what could possibly be "wrong" with me, we simply did the tests they would have had us do for fertility treatment, and let nature take its course.

The following are some of the first steps that a fertility clinic would take in determining your level of fertility and the course of action to take. You can do all of this for a few hundred dollars. Be sure and keep all of your results to take with you if you do ever end up throwing down the approximately $5000 it takes to start up fertility services.

Sperm count and motility.

First, after six months of charting my temperatures and being fairly certain that we had nailed ovulation each month, we had my husband's sperm count checked. This wasn't as easy as it sounds. There is only one place in my hometown that will let you walk in with a prescription from your GP for a sperm analysis. Call your GP and see where they tell you to go.

Blood work.

When the sperm proved themselves worthy, I then had my blood work done, mainly to see if my hormone levels were where they should be to maintain a pregnancy. (**Make sure you check your progesterone levels during the *second* phase of your cycle, meaning after ovulation** – that's when you need high progesterone to hold a pregnancy). My midwife did all these tests for a fraction of the cost of a doctor.

Ultrasound.

I also had a pelvic ultrasound to see if my uterus and ovaries appeared healthy and normal.

The next step would have been to find out if my vaginal secretions were killing my husband's sperm. They do this by swabbing your vagina just after sex and seeing how many of the little guys are still swimming. This is invasive, and while I was putting it off, we conceived. And I have to add, just like everyone said would happen, we conceived during one of the two months we had taken "off" from trying. I wasn't even charting (slap my wrist). It was just what Nature had in mind.

I've heard that after age 35, couples have only a 15% chance of conceiving every month. Bearing that in mind, realize that it just might take a while. However, your eggs are getting older every month, and if you're just dying to give birth and can afford both financially and emotionally to do the fertility thing, it is an option.

If you want to conceive (or avoid pregnancy), spend $30 on Toni's book instead of $30,000 on a fertility doctor. If you end up needing the fertility doctor, you'll at least know your body and when you tend to ovulate, which is something no doctor can know.

- Chapter 23 -
Hormone Imbalances, Toxic Bodies, PCOS, and My Story

There are many physiological reasons for infertility, such as endometriosis, a lack of viable eggs, a blocked fallopian tube, or a low sperm count. If you don't think you have any problems and you're simply having trouble conceiving, you either don't know when you're fertile, or you've probably just got hormones that are out of whack.

If you suspect hormonal issues, welcome to my world and to the world of most people in western society today. I can't tell you, though, how grateful I am to my wacky hormones for prodding me into taking my health into my own hands.

In our life times, most of us have eaten or have drunk mass quantities of hormones found in our meat and dairy products. These hormones, along with sugar, fried food, red meat and dairy fat, cause us to develop hormone imbalances and to produce an over-abundance of estrogen.

"High fats mean high circulating estrogen. Too much estrogen is the most common cause of cysts."[1] Under normal dietary circumstances, say around 200 years ago, the human body experienced a glorious, magical, usually perfect hormonal symphony over the course of its lifetime. We are only beginning to understand the extent of the dialogue between our hormones and our health, but we do know that when hormones get messed up, people get really messed up.

Take for instance when someone has a genetic predisposition for too much or too little growth hormone to be produced. At some point, for normal people, around the age of 23, our growth hormone stops being produced. For "giants" this never happens. They keep growing and growing for the rest of their lives. This is just a highly visible example of wacky hormones.

Hormone imbalance is sad and scary. Athletes who take HGH (Human Growth Hormone) must be out of their brawny little minds.

My Story

When I was trying to conceive my first child, I was seeing an acupuncturist because I knew that acupuncture had a good track record for fertility. One of the things that became apparent as we were paying close attention to my cycles was that I was spotting mid-cycle right around ovulation. This can be a totally normal occurrence; however, I had had a miscarriage three years before, and I wanted to rule out that there might still be some fetal tissue in my uterus.

This was my own idea, and I couldn't get it out of my head.

So, I went to the OBGYN, but only for an ultrasound. I get my well-woman exams from a midwife and I actually love them. (See Introduction.) The good doctor greased up my belly and had a peek. After a minute or two, he says, "Well, the good news is your uterus looks great. Nothing suspicious is going on in there. The bad news, however, is that your right ovary is the size of a grapefruit. Look here, you see those little cysts that look like little peas? They're bloating up your ovary."

I said, "What do you recommend?"

He said, "That we take the ovary."

I replied, "I truly believe in the body's ability to heal itself. I want to do acupuncture and Reiki and look into what could be causing this nutritionally before I just sign up for surgery. How long before it has to come out?"

He originally said to come back in four weeks, but when he thought a little longer, knowing that I was paying for these visits out of pocket, he said to make it four months.

I immediately came home and opened up *Healthy Healing* by Linda Page. I looked up the section on ovaries. And there it was in black and white, the exact description of my ovary puffed up with little corpora lutea, the little egg sacs that are supposed to be re-absorbed by the body each month after it pushes the egg out of the ovary.

She called my condition "Polycystic Ovarian Syndrome" or PCOS. She said it's usually caused by a hormonal imbalance and can have many symptoms including infertility. She told me cut out red meat, dairy, and coffee. I did this. I also got my acupuncturist to treat it. She gave me moxa, a Chinese herb, to burn over my ovaries daily to help "move" the masses in the area. I performed Reiki on myself daily as well. I visualized healthy, happy, functional ovaries.

~ ~ ~ ~ ~

When I went back four months later to actually see the ovary again, lo and behold, it was absolutely normal. I love that the good doctor could show me my insides. I don't love that his only solution was to surgically remove the beacon of my lack of health.

Basically, if you're having trouble conceiving, you very likely have a hormonal imbalance or you're just too toxic to conceive. Susun Weed's book, *Wise Woman Herbal for the Childbearing Year*, discusses the importance of getting your body ready for pregnancy. It's simply a matter of making healthy decisions. The healthier you are, the more likely you are to have a successful pregnancy. Start taking care of yourself, see an acupuncturist, get Linda Page's book, and hopefully get pregnant.

- Chapter 24 -
Acupuncture, Herbs, and Healthy Eating

I am 100% certain that acupuncture and the herbs that my acupuncturist gave me not only helped me become pregnant, but also helped me maintain the pregnancy.

Acupuncture and herbs balance your hormones and tonify your reproductive system.

Acupuncturists also tell you what foods to eat to get your particular body balanced. If your kidney chi or liver chi is weak, they might recommend that you eat more bright, rainbow-colored vegetables like beets, carrots, and greens.

If your blood is deficient, they might recommend that you eat blood-building foods like black beans, raisins, and organic, hormone-free red meat in moderation. An acupuncturist will not only treat you, but also will help tailor a regimen suited to your particular well being. You will learn more about creating vibrant health from a good acupuncturist than from anyone else. Get some good references for an acupuncturist. This is not someone I would look for in the yellow pages.

Black beans are a highly recommended food for promoting fertility. It is also recommended that you eat organic meat, poultry and wild-caught seafood, as those conventionally farmed are fed genetically modified grains. Avoid GMO's now and for the rest of your life.

There is also an herbal supplement you might look into taking called Vitex or Chaste Tree. It enhances fertility over time. It works best over the course of a year or two.

An excellent book to use as a resource is Paul Pitchford's *Healing with Whole Foods*.

- Chapter 25 -

Miscarriage:

How to Have One at Home and Not Freak Out

First of all, miscarriage is nature's way of taking care of things that really weren't meant to be.

It's possible, though, that sometimes miscarriages might be avoidable. For instance, if you're prone to low progesterone levels (yet another hormone balancing issue,) it might be hard for you to develop and keep a pregnancy. If you experience multiple miscarriages, I would most definitely see a referred acupuncturist.

Women have had miscarriages since there were women. In fact, I have a sister-in-law who had four. Some women never experience it, while other women, it seems, get more than their fair share. Either way, it's an entirely normal and natural experience that you don't need to freak out about.

Sometimes, a fetus isn't developing properly, and Nature knows what She's doing. It's really something to be grateful for.

It's never easy. My first pregnancy ended in miscarriage.

People don't really talk about it. It's not the most pleasant of topics, but I don't mind talking about it at all. So here goes. Miscarriage is like labor, but it sucks. It's like 50% of what having a baby is with no prize at the end, just an empty, sad feeling.

What to Do

When you're having a miscarriage, you basically are in labor. Your uterus contracts just like during labor to expel the fetus. It's painful like childbirth, but you bleed much more. Actually in childbirth, there's usually not much blood. A miscarriage is somewhere between a really crampy period and labor.

Hopefully, you'll have been visiting a midwife during your pregnancy, and if you start to miscarry, you can call her. She'll hold your hand and coach you through it over the phone.

At the same time, send someone to the local herb shop to pick up some blue and black cohosh tinctures. They induce labor and help to expel the fetus.

One thing to watch for is how much blood there is. If you're filling more than one pad an hour, you could possibly be hemorrhaging, and that's when you'd need some medical assistance. Otherwise, you're absolutely fine just staying at home for the duration.

The other thing to watch for, graphic, but important, is a small piece of fleshy tissue that will look something like chicken. You need to make sure that this passes. It was the fetus that wasn't developing. If the fetus had been developing somewhat properly, it might look more like a little fetus. Either way, when this passes, you'll know that you most likely don't need a DNC, which stands for dilation and curettage and means uterus scraping. This procedure is to be avoided if unnecessary because complications include puncture of the uterus, tear of the cervix, scarring of the uterine lining, and infection.[2]

A warm bath is most helpful when it comes to easing the pain of the contractions. In fact, every time I got in the tub, my contractions would miraculously stop. I still had the miscarriage, but was ever grateful for that bathtub.

Also, my husband never left my side during the miscarriage, which lasted around 8-10 hours. I needed his support. I was extremely emotional before, during, and after the miscarriage.

This is to be expected, due to all the hormones doing the tag team thing. The hormones that keep you pregnant come to a screeching halt and tag off to Team Oxytocin, which kicks labor in.

In fact, it happens so fast that miscarriage seemed 50 times more emotional than birth itself.

If you have a miscarriage, just remember all of the billions of women throughout history who have experienced it.

Don't go into a place of fear. You can do it. You will feel a loss, but it was a little life that wasn't meant to be. And no matter how sad you feel, time will pass.

And time does heal.

- Afterward -

No matter how you give birth, especially if you have a C-section or a full-on epidural, pitocin and the works, the person you were when you were pregnant and the mother you are to your child are by far the most important things. I know a mother who came from a family of homebirthers, but ended up having to give birth to her two children by cesarean. She brought to my attention that birth is only one day and your relationship with your child is a lifetime. I am in 100% agreement with this statement. However, it just so happens that that one day can be such a powerful, gentle and memorable one.

What's more important – a healthy, happy marriage or a great wedding? Obviously, the marriage itself is far more important than the wedding. But a wedding happens to be an opportunity for the sacred to be experienced and remembered. It's the same with birth. In the great scheme of things, birth is just one day. But it was such an amazing day for me, my husband, my mother, and my sons, that I wanted to share it with you and make it a possibility for more families.

I received a card after the birth of my first son. On the front was a drawing of a cute mama bear holding a new little baby bear in bed with her. The inside of the card read, "Love is a Homebirth." I hope one day you get the opportunity to understand.

- About the Author -

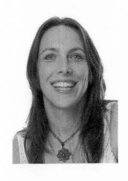

Betsy Dewey is a musician, teacher, business woman, writer, and free-thinker. With degrees from both Vanderbilt University and The University of North Carolina, she is a natural born communicator who especially enjoys sharing her experiences and growing knowledge about pregnancy, homebirth, natural living, parenting, etc. with those who might benefit.

This is her debut book, a milestone, a first among more to come. You can stay informed by visiting www.betsydewey.com.

Betsy enjoys writing from home, raising her two young boys and living life fully as a family with her husband.

- Appendix -

Supplemental Reading

The following is a list of books that I highly recommend. Many of them are mentioned in this book:

Early Start Potty Training – Linda Sonna

The EverythingToddler Activities Book – Joni Levine

Feed Me I'm Yours – Vicki Lansky

The Fertility Diet – Jorge E. Chavarro and Walter C. Willette

Healing With Whole Foods – Paul Pitchford

How to Have a Smarter Baby – Susan Ludington-Hoe

Loving Hands: The Traditional Art of Baby Massage – Frederick Leboyer

The Nursing Mother's Guide to Weaning – Huggins and Ziedrich

The Psychology of Achievement (CD's) – Brian Tracy

Seat of the Soul – Gary Zukav

The Secret Life of the Unborn Child – Thomas Verny

Smart Medicine for a Healthier Child – Janet Zand, Robert Rountree, and Rachel Walton

Super Baby Food – Ruth Yaron

Taking Charge of Your Fertility – Toni Weschler

The Vaccine Book: Making the Right Decision for Your Child - Dr. Robert Sears

Wise Woman Herbal for the Childbearing Year – Susun Weed

You are your Child's First Teacher – Rahima Baldwin

Nurtured by Love - Dr. Shinichi Suzuki

Ability Development From Age Zero - Dr. Shinichi Suzuki

Journeying Through Pregnancy and Birth – meditation CD distributed by:

> WomanWay
>
> 1081 High Falls Rd.
>
> Catskill, NY 12414
>
> (866)205-5004 (pin#1212)

Awesome Children's CDs

(or CDs that won't drive you crazy by the time you've heard them 100 times.)

> *Indian Elephant Tea* by the Big Kidz Band
>
> *Dreamland* by Putumayo (anything by Putumayo kids)
>
> Raffi - all of them
>
> *The Biscuit Brothers* – all of them
>
> *Suzuki Violin* Volumes 1-4

Baby Genius – Children's Songs

Reggae for Kids – RAS records

Short and Sweet by Jimmy Magoo

Washboard Jungle

Color Wheel Cartwheel - Laura Freeman

Online Resources:

BetsyDewey.com - This is my website filled with tidbits of musefruit relating to everything childbirth, parenting, life and freedom. Please visit often, subscribe to my posts, and leave comments or questions. I look forward to meeting you.

Mothering Magazine is the premier, leading-edge on-line publication for conscious parenting for both fathers and mothers. The articles are open-minded, well-researched and well-documented. Topics cover everything from circumcision to autism. The advertising in the magazine is naturally based, from organic cotton diapers to natural, wooden toys. I have learned more about parenting from this magazine than from any other source excluding my own parents.

I learned how to respond to people when they asked if I was ever going to wean my two year old. "Oh, we'll probably have him weaned by the time he goes off to college," is a good one. I also learned that this was none of their business. If you're making parenting decisions that you feel are unquestionably the best decisions for your child, but they're still a little eccentric or ahead of their time, this magazine provides a community of other parents who are in the same boat. If you question the over-use of vaccinations, disposable diapers, formula, and letting babies "cry it out," you will love this publication.

I truly believe it to be indispensable for parents in today's world. The reason I say to start subscribing while you're pregnant is that you're going to want to know that plastic baby bottles might be leaching PVC or BPA into whatever your baby consumes from them before you buy all your bottles. You're going to want to know about the harsh reality of circumcision before you do it. You're going to want to know everything this magazine brings up before the stork shows up. I didn't end up with a stack of old Mothering Magazines, hence learning of its existence, until my baby was 6 months old. I poured over the information therein and only wished I had gotten word of it a year before. So, to quote Vanilla Ice – word to your mother.

- Bibliography -

i Linda Page, Healthy Healing, 11th ed. (Traditional Wisdom, Inc, 2003), 471.

ii Medline Plus Medical Encyclopedia, "D and C," Medline Plus, http://www.nlmmih.gov/medlineplus/ency/article/002914.html (accessed Jn. 8, 2009)

iii Ina May Gaskin, "Masking Maternal Mortality," Mothering Magazine, March-April 2008, 66.

iv NationMaster, "Health Statistics > Maternal mortality (most recent) by country," NationMaster,

http://www.nationmaster.com/graph/hea_mat_mor-health-maternal-mortality (accessed Sept. 23, 2008).

v (Texas Lay midwifery Program, Six Year Report, 1983- 1989, Bernstein & Bryant, Appendix Vlllf, Texas Department of Health, 1100 West 49th St., Austin, TX 78756-3199.)

vi Jan Poorter, Primary Health Care in the Netherlands, Ministry of Health, Welfare and Sport (The Hague: January 2005): 31; www.minvws.nl/en/folders/cz/2005/primary-health-care.asp (accessed Sept. 23, 2008).

vii Geography IQ, "Rankings > Infant mortality rate," Geography IQ, http://www.geographyiq.com/ranking/ranking_Infant_Mortality_Rate_aall.htm (accessed Sept. 23, 2008).

viii NationMaster, "Health Statistics > Maternal mortality (most recent) by country," NationMaster, http://www.nationmaster.com/graph/hea_mat_mor-health-maternal-mortality (accessed Sept. 23, 2008).

ix Linda T. Kohn, Janet M. Corrigan, and Molla S. Donaldson, To Err is Human: Building a Safer Health System. (The National Academies Press, 2000),1. http://www.nap.edu/openbook.php?record_id=9728&page=1 (accessed Sept. 17,2008).

x Wendy Ponte, "Cesarean Birth in a Culture of Fear," Mothering Magazine, September-October 2007,50.

xi Ibid.,53.

xii *Harvard Health Publications*, "Amniocentesis," Harvard Medical School, http://www.health.harvard.edu/diagnostic-tests/amniosentesis.htm (accessed Aug 27, 2008).

xiii About.com, "Incidence of Down Syndrome with Increasing Maternal Age," The New York Times Companny, http://pregnancy.about.com/cs/downsyndrome/l/bldownssyn.htm (accessed Apr 20, 2009).

xiv Susan W. Enouen, "Down Syndrome and Abortion," (Christian Life Resources Inc) www.christianliferesources.com/?library/view.php&articleid=1254 (accessed May 11, 2009).

xv UNFPA, "Maternal Mortality Figures Show Limited Progress in Making Motherhood Safer," United Nations Population Fund, http://www.unfpa.org/mothers/statistics.htm (accessed Sept. 17, 2008).

xvi Raven Lang, *The Birth Book*, 1972.

xvii Thomas Verny and John Kelly, *The Secret Life of the Unborn Child*. (New York: Dell Publishing, 1981),16.

xviii Julie Bouchet Horowitz, "A Special Gift: Breastfeeding an Adopted Baby," Mothering Magazine, January-February 2001, 62.

xix Oregon.gov Health and Human Services, "The Benefits of Breastfeeding," Oregon.gov, http://www.oregon.gov/DHS/ph/bf/benefits.shtml#long-baby (accessed Sept. 23, 2008).

xx Ibid.

xxi *The Stork Cloth Diaper Service*, "Which are Better, Cloth or Disposable Diapers?" The Stork Cloth Diaper Service, http://www.thestork.biz/truths.html (accessed Sept. 1, 2008).

xxii Environmental Working Group, "Body Burden - The Pollution in Newborns," Environmental Working Group, http:// archive.ewg.org/reports/bodyburden2/execsumm.php (accessed Sept. 1, 2008).

xxiii PR Web Press Release Newswire, "Doctors' Mistakes Causing Penile Damage," Vocus PRW Holdings, LLC, http:// www.prweb.com/releases/2002/7/prweb42218.htm (accessed Sept. 1, 2008).

xxiv American Academy of Pediatrics Task Force on Circumcision, "PEDIATRICS Vol. 103 No. 3 March 1999, pp. 686-693 AMERICAN ACADEMY OF PEDIATRICS: Circumcision Policy Statement," American Academy of Pediatrics, http:// aappolicy.aappublications.org/cgi/content/full/pediatrics; 103/3/686 (accessed Sept. 1, 2008).

xxv Doctors Opposing Circumcision, website home page, www.doctorsopposingcircumcision.org. (accessed Sept. 1, 2008).

xxvi The Circumcision Reference Library, "United States Circumcision Incidence," The Circumcision Reference Library, www.cirp.org/library/statistics/USA/ (accessed Sept. 1, 2008).

xxvii Gussie Fauntleroy, "The Truth About Circumcision and HIV," Mothering Magazine, July-August 2008,48.

xxviii Environmental Working Group, "Body Burden - The Pollution in Newborns," Environmental Working Group, http:// archive.ewg.org/reports/bodyburden2/execsumm.php (accessed Sept. 1, 2008).

Made in the USA
Charleston, SC
11 September 2011